STUDY GUIDE for
PATHOPHYSIOLOGY

STUDY GUIDE for
COPSTEAD & BANASIK
PATHOPHYSIOLOGY

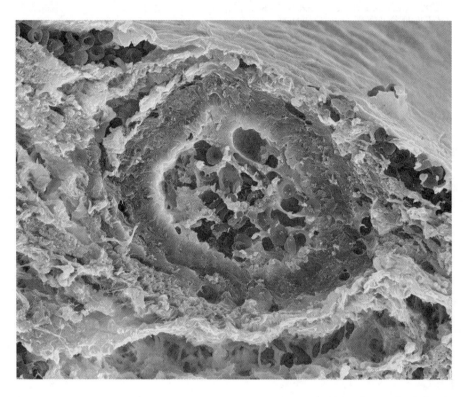

THIRD EDITION

PREPARED BY
JACQUELYN L. BANASIK, PhD, ARNP

Associate Professor
WSU Intercollegiate College of Nursing
Washington State University
Spokane, Washington

ROBERTA J. EMERSON, PhD, CCRN

Associate Professor
WSU Intercollegiate College of Nursing
Washington State University
Spokane, Washington

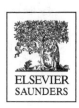

ELSEVIER
SAUNDERS

ELSEVIER
SAUNDERS

11830 Westline Industrial Drive
St. Louis, Missouri 63146

STUDY GUIDE FOR COPSTEAD & BANASIK:
PATHOPHYSIOLOGY, THIRD EDITION

NOTICE

Pathophysiology is an ever-changing field. Standard safety precautions must be followed, but as new research and clinical experience broaden our knowledge, changes in treatment and drug therapy may become necessary or appropriate. Readers are advised to check the most current product information provided by the manufacturer of each drug to be administered to verify the recommended dose, the method and duration of administration, and contraindications. It is the responsibility of the licensed prescriber, relying on experience and knowledge of the patient, to determine dosages and the best treatment for each individual patient. Neither the publisher nor the author assumes any liability for any injury and/or damage to persons or property arising from this publication.

ISBN-13: 978-1-4160-2383-8
ISBN-10: 1-4160-2383-6

Executive Publisher: Darlene Como
Managing Editor: Brian Dennison
Developmental Editor: Barbara Watts
Editorial Assistant: Katherine V. Judge
Publishing Services Manager: Deborah L. Vogel
Project Manager: Deon Lee
Design Manager: Teresa McBryan

Printed in the United States of America

Last digit is the print number: 9   8   7   6   5   4   3   2

Preface

Pathophysiology is a complex and ever-expanding subject. In an effort to provide students with a comprehensive reference, most pathophysiology texts contain a seemingly overwhelming amount of information, facts, and details. The Copstead & Banasik text *Pathophysiology,* Third Edition, includes Key Questions and Key Concepts to help the student focus on the important points. This workbook builds on that approach by providing review questions that correspond to the main ideas presented in each unit of the textbook. Many students of pathophysiology are uncertain of the adequacy of their knowledge, even after they have read and studied,

particularly as examination time draws near. This student Study Guide is designed to facilitate a focus on the important concepts and to help students build confidence in their knowledge base and test-taking skills.

Although this workbook follows the organization of the Copstead & Banasik textbook, it also can be used in the context of other courses or as a refresher before taking the NCLEX® examination.

We hope you find it useful.

Jacquelyn L. Banasik
Roberta J. Emerson

Contents

Keys to Success

While the amount of information contained in a typical pathophysiology text is daunting, a number of strategies will help you grasp the underlying concepts and therefore be able to retain the information and apply it. For many students, nursing school provides at least one educational challenge they have not experienced previously: the need to apply knowledge learned in various theory classes to their patients in the clinical setting. Relying on old techniques of memorizing for examinations and then moving on to the next topic will no longer work. Your theory classes may not have comprehensive examinations, but your clinical practice surely will require that previous knowledge be retained and applied in a variety of situations. This is not to say that you will not need to memorize some things, but rather that you need to know why you are memorizing and how these memorized facts will help you sort out assessment findings in clinical practice situations.

KEEP YOUR PURPOSE IN MIND

Before setting out to study pathophysiology, it is helpful to think about the purpose for knowing this information. This will help you focus on main points. Nurses use pathophysiology for three main purposes:

1. *To predict the clinical manifestations likely to be present in a patient with a known medical diagnosis.* This allows the nurse to tailor assessment of the patient and to monitor signs and symptoms that indicate whether the patient is improving or getting worse. Assessment findings that do not seem to fit with the patient's diagnosis can also be recognized and investigated.

2. *To formulate hypotheses about the meaning of clinical findings and their etiology.* Each pathophysiologic process has characteristic or typical manifestations that usually accompany it. One finding is seldom enough to lead to a diagnosis; rather, it is a constellation of findings that indicates a problem. Manifestations often vary somewhat from person to person, making the detective work more difficult. Because of their close contact with patients, nurses are often first to suspect a pathologic problem in a patient. A good understanding of pathophysiology allows early recognition and initiation of therapy. For example, the findings of fever, increased respiratory rate, shallow breathing, and adventitious breath sounds in a postoperative patient may indicate the development of hypostatic pneumonia. An astute nurse can intervene early and reduce morbidity.

3. *To evaluate the appropriateness of prescribed therapies and assess for possible contraindications.* The pathophysiologic mechanisms of particular disease processes usually imply which treatment may be effective and which may be contraindicated. For example, a patient with coronary heart disease may appropriately be prescribed a β-adrenergic blocking drug to reduce cardiac workload, but if the patient also has asthma, the drug may exacerbate bronchospasm. This indicates that either the respiratory system response should be monitored or perhaps the prescription should be questioned.

Thus, it is helpful to ask yourself how the information you are reading in the text will be applied clinically. This technique will keep you focused on the important points and also provide a motivation for learning the material; a patient will be depending on your knowledge base. Few things are more satisfying in clinical practice than diagnosing a problem early and preventing a patient from experiencing serious consequences. In this regard, the application of pathophysiology is a rewarding kind of detective work—and it is fun to solve the case!

APPLY PATHOPHYSIOLOGY TO LIFE

Pathophysiology is everywhere! Conversations with your next-door neighbor, complaints from your family members, and medical dramas on television provide wonderful practice in honing your assessment and diagnostic skills. Try to analyze the signs you observe, and predict a diagnosis—before the television episode reveals the answer. (Do not, however, dispense your medical opinion. That will get you into big trouble. This is just an exercise of the mind.)

When you begin your first clinical rotation, you will have opportunities to apply your knowledge in real situations. Although it is natural to focus on tasks and on learning to communicate with patients, be sure to spend some focused time trying to understand your patient's pathophysiology. Look up the labs. Note the physical signs and symptoms. Try to correlate these with the medical diagnosis. Look over the medications to determine whether they make sense with regard to the diagnosis. Ask your clinical instructor questions when you are not sure. (Do not be afraid of showing your ignorance. Clinical instructors generally appreciate a curious student!) Take every available opportunity to apply the concepts you are learning in your pathophysiology course.

KNOW THE RELEVANT ANATOMY AND PHYSIOLOGY

Students who have a good grasp on anatomy and physiology (A&P) tend to have an easier time understanding pathophysiology. Conversely, students who are no longer facile with A&P are likely to struggle and find that they must review the normal structures and functions before they can proceed. The Copstead & Banasik textbook incorporates this review into each unit. The best place to start learning pathophysiology is to get A&P into your working knowledge. Each unit in this Study Guide begins with exercises to help you test your A&P knowledge. If this section does not come easy, you will benefit from reading the review chapter in the text. The importance of a good basis in A&P cannot be overemphasized!

DEVELOP GOOD STUDY SKILLS

Depending on your learning style, you may find one or more of the following general study tips to be helpful:

- Read with a purpose. Use the *Key Questions* to help you focus on major concepts as you read. Use the *Key Concepts* sections in each chapter to review what you have read and test your understanding.
- Pay attention to new words. Vocabulary is a major part of learning new content; pathophysiology has its own language, and you need to learn it. There is a glossary at the back of the textbook to help you.
- Memorize what you must, like the normal values for arterial blood gases. But think through the application so that you understand it (why *does* pH go down when P_{CO_2} goes up?).
- Put facts into patterns. Sometimes the patterns are obvious; other times, you have to create them. Mnemonics are helpful to remember some things, like the order of the cranial nerves.

- Put what you have read into your own words. If you can explain concepts to someone else so that he or she understands it, you know you really understand it yourself!
- Do not forget that pathophysiology predicts presentation. When you feel you understand the pathophysiology, make a list of the likely signs and symptoms that the abnormality suggests. Then go back and check your thinking. It is better to be able to figure out the clinical manifestations as predicted by the underlying mechanisms than it is to memorize them.
- Recognize how you learn best. Some people learn well by reading information. Others find listening is better for them, and reading aloud and listening to tape recordings of classes is best. Some people make drawings or "trees" showing relationships of ideas.
- Repeat, review, and rest. A single study period will not lock content into your long-term memory. Go over the content area again, checking the accuracy of your recall. Prolonged study periods

are not productive; you actually begin to lose efficiency. Do not try to study for more than an hour at a time without a 10- or 15-minute break.

- Try a group review session. Many students find this to be helpful in checking their thinking and preparing for examinations. All participants should have studied the material already. Use the time as a question-and-answer session. Do not rely on notes; try to answer from memory. The *Key Questions* and *Key Concepts* from the text can be used as a guide for formulating quiz questions—or adapt questions from this Study Guide.

USE THE STUDY GUIDE TO TEST YOURSELF

After you have read and studied, answer the pathophysiology questions provided in this Study Guide. It is best to take the entire examination all at once. Make yourself commit to the answers before you check the key. This will help you be a better test taker. Even if you do not think you know the answer to a question, you may be able to figure it out. Sometimes the only way to the correct answer is through recognition of the incorrect answers. Score yourself and review the incorrect answers. Is the answer obvious to you now that you see it? If so, you probably understand the concepts adequately, but you are misreading questions or reading things into the answers. Alternatively, you may not have spent enough time getting the information into your "working knowledge" and had trouble with retrieval. More study time is indicated. If you do not understand the question even after seeing the right answer, you need to go back to the chapter and reread the content until you can see that the right answer is right. Your ability to focus on the important material will help you improve your test-taking skills with time. Enjoy the challenge!

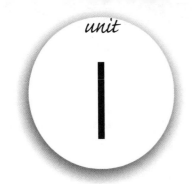

unit

1

Pathophysiologic Processes

Chapters 1 and 2

NORMAL ANATOMY AND PHYSIOLOGY REVIEW
True/False

Indicate whether the following statements regarding the anatomy and physiology of homeostasis and stress responses are true (T) or false (F).

1. _____ Homeostasis is a physiologic condition in which all systems are functioning at the ideal.

2. _____ Most homeostatic feedback mechanisms function on the principle of negative feedback.

3. _____ Homeostatic mechanisms are initiated as soon as disease becomes clinically evident.

4. _____ The normal ranges for physiologic parameters such as blood pressure, blood electrolyte levels, and other laboratory tests will vary according to the population studied.

5. _____ Trends and changes in an individual's laboratory values are more reliable than a single observation.

6. _____ Most of the signs and symptoms of an acute response to stress are attributable to activation of the sympathetic nervous system.

7. _____ Adaptation to stress is unsuccessful when homeostasis is not maintained or restored.

8. _____ Selye's three phases of the stress response include alarm, initiation, and resistance.

9. _____ Cortisol is released during the stress response and serves to make more glucose available to the brain.

10. _____ Antidiuretic hormone is released during stress and serves to increase urine output and reduce blood pressure.

PATHOPHYSIOLOGY QUESTIONS
True/False

Indicate whether the following statements regarding the pathophysiology of homeostasis and stress responses are true (T) or false (F).

11. _____ There is usually a single, well-defined cause or etiologic factor for a disease process.

12. _____ Pathogenesis refers to the mechanisms whereby an etiologic factor leads to the typically observed clinical manifestations of a disease.

13. _____ Manifestations of a disease process vary among individuals.

14. _____ Epidemiology is the study of patterns of disease among human populations.

15. _____ The principal utility of epidemiology is to determine the best way to manage a disease after it occurs in an individual.

16. _____ Hyperplasia of the adrenal cortex, lymphoid atrophy, and stomach ulceration are features of the general adaptation syndrome.

17. _____ The excessive release of cortisol in response to prolonged or poorly adapted stress serves to suppress the immune system.

18. _____ Although the CNS is known to affect the immune system through various neurotransmitters, the immune system does not affect the CNS.

19. _____ Most individuals will respond to an identical stressful situation in a similar physiologic manner.

20. _____ A means of coping with stress is considered functional if it alleviates the subjective feeling of stress even though it does not necessarily resolve the stressful situation.

Compare/Contrast

The stress response has been implicated in the pathogenesis of many disorders and disease processes in humans. For each of the physiologic systems below, list three to five disorders that are thought to have a significant stress component.

Physiologic System	Stress-Induced Disease Process
Nervous system	
Cardiovascular system	
Gastrointestinal system	
Genitourinary system	
Integumentary system	
Respiratory system	
Immune system	
Endocrine system	
Musculoskeletal system	

Multiple Choice

Select the one best answer to each of the following questions.

21. Pathophysiology includes all of the following elements except:
    A. etiology.
    B. clinical manifestations.
    C. mechanisms of pathogenesis.
    D. clinical management.

22. Acquired immunodeficiency syndrome (AIDS) is a disorder in which immune cells are infected with human immunodeficiency virus (HIV) and are subsequently destroyed, leading to increased susceptibility to opportunistic infections. What is the *etiologic* factor in AIDS?
    A. Increased susceptibility to opportunistic infections
    B. Destruction of immune cells
    C. HIV virus
    D. Acquired immunodeficiency syndrome

23. Understanding the epidemiologic progression of a disease is essential for effective:
    A. prevention.
    B. detection.
    C. treatment.
    D. monitoring.

24. Which of the following is an example of primary prevention?
    A. Childhood immunization for communicable diseases
    B. Routine PAP smear of the cervix
    C. Amniocentesis to detect genetic abnormality in the fetus
    D. Range-of-motion exercises to prevent disuse atrophy in the stroke patient

25. Which of the following findings would indicate that a patient may be experiencing a "fight or flight" reaction to a stressor?
    A. Constricted pupils
    B. Flushed face
    C. Increased heart rate
    D. Frequent sighing or yawning

26. Which of Selye's stages of stress response is a patient in if he is experiencing gastrointestinal bleeding secondary to peptic ulcer disease?
    A. Alarm
    B. Resistance
    C. Exhaustion
    D. Illness

27. A stressor that stimulates the release of endorphins in the CNS is likely to be interpreted as:
    A. pleasurable.
    B. painful.
    C. unimportant.
    D. noxious.

28. Several hormones are released during stress that serve to increase blood glucose levels. These include all of the following except:
    A. cortisol.
    B. growth hormone.
    C. epinephrine.
    D. testosterone.

29. Indicators that a person who is experiencing stress has achieved resistance include:
    A. increased glucocorticoid secretion.
    B. sympathetic activity returning to baseline.
    C. fight-or-flight reaction maintaining homeostasis.
    D. absence of catecholamine secretion.

30. Behavioral indicators that coping is ineffective include all of the following except:
    A. sleeping more.
    B. major depression.
    C. inability to concentrate.
    D. anorexia.

Fill in the Blank

Fill in the blanks with the appropriate word or words.

31. Serum levels of cortisol fluctuate over a 24-hour period reflecting a _____ _____, also known as _____ _____.

32. Visiting a hospital in another state, differences in laboratory values are seen because they are based on different _____.

33. The specific cause of some diseases, such as essential hypertension, is unknown, so these conditions are called _____.

34. An undesirable condition that develops following treatment is called _____.

35. The three major body systems involved in the stress response are the _____, _____, and _____ systems.

36. The release of two steroid hormones _____ and _____ occurs in the resistance stage of the general adaptation syndrome.

37. The hormone that provides the key link between stress and the immune system is _____.

38. The local adaptation syndrome corresponds to the _____ response.

39. The biopsychosocial process of thinking and acting in a stressful situation is called _____, whereas _____ is the process of change that occurs in response to altered circumstances.

40. _____ are chemicals released by the brain that cause euphoria, sedation, and elevation of the pain threshold.

Case Studies

Marge is a 42-year-old woman who works full time as a legal secretary and has three children, ages 6, 9, and 11. She was divorced 6 months ago and relocated to a new school district. Her children are adjusting to school, but Marge has not established any friendships in the neighborhood. She is in the clinic today with a severe migraine headache that has not responded to her usual ibuprofen medications.

41. According to Selye, since Marge is experiencing headaches and is seeking medical care, she is in the stage of:
    A. alarm.
    B. resistance.
    C. exhaustion.
    D. symptom emergence.

42. Since stress is believed to be a significant factor in the etiologic progression of migraine headache, it may be helpful for Marge to:
    A. avoid medicating her headaches.
    B. eliminate stressful situations.
    C. cope more effectively.
    D. identify precipitating stressors and initiate preventive measures.

43. Marge indicates that she does not think her migraines are a result of stress because her sister is in a much worse life situation than she is and does not get migraines. Which of the following statements is the best basis for a reply?
    A. Perhaps your sister's situation is not as bad as you think it is.
    B. People respond to stressful situations in different ways.
    C. Migraines are always stress related.
    D. Perhaps your sister has better coping skills.

Jean is a 28-year-old woman with chronic back pain subsequent to a motor vehicle accident she suffered at age 22. She is currently in the hospital in preparation for back surgery the next day.

44. The nursing aide caring for Jean reports that Jean does not seem to be too stressed because her vital signs are normal and she is sitting quietly in bed. Which of the following statements is the best basis for a reply?
    A. People with chronic stress due to pain may not exhibit a sympathetic response when stressed.
    B. She is not stressed because the surgery is going to help her pain.
    C. She probably has better coping skills than other people because she has been in pain so long.
    D. The pain medication for her back probably takes care of her stress.

45. Jean's preoperative laboratory tests show a slightly elevated blood glucose level. This may be attributed to:
    A. her NPO (nothing by mouth) status prior to surgery.
    B. increased cortisol release in response to stress.
    C. decreased physical activity while in the hospital.
    D. a side effect of her pain medication.

46. Jean indicates that she would like the television to be turned on to distract her from thinking about the upcoming surgery. This is an example of:
    A. ineffective coping.
    B. Selye's stage of exhaustion.
    C. resolving the stressor.
    D. functional coping.

ANSWER KEY

NORMAL ANATOMY AND PHYSIOLOGY REVIEW
True/False

1. F
2. T
3. F
4. T
5. T
6. T
7. T
8. F
9. T
10. F

PATHOPHYSIOLOGY QUESTIONS
True/False

11. F
12. T
13. T
14. T
15. F
16. T
17. T
18. F
19. F
20. T

Compare/Contrast

(See textbook Figure 2-13 for more examples.)

Physiologic System	Stress-Induced Disease Process
Nervous system	Nervous tic; fatigue; anxiety; depression; insomnia; headaches
Cardiovascular system	Abnormal heart rate, rhythm; hypertension; stroke; coronary heart disease
Gastrointestinal system	Gastritis; irritable bowel syndrome; ulcerative colitis; Crohn disease
Genitourinary system	Irritable bladder; impotence; frigidity; menstrual irregularity
Integumentary system	Hair loss; rashes
Respiratory system	Hyperventilation; asthma; frequent upper respiratory infections
Immune system	Immune deficiency; autoimmune disease; frequent infections
Endocrine system	Hyperglycemia; diabetes mellitus
Musculoskeletal system	Muscle tension headache; backache; autoimmune and inflammatory joint disorders; fibromyalgia

Multiple Choice

21. D
22. C
23. A
24. A
25. C
26. C
27. A
28. D
29. B
30. A

Fill in the Blank

31. circadian rhythm; diurnal variation
32. populations
33. idiopathic
34. iatrogenic
35. nervous, endocrine, immune
36. cortisol, aldosterone
37. cortisol
38. inflammatory
39. coping; adaptation
40. endorphins

Case Studies

41. C
42. D
43. B
44. A
45. B
46. D

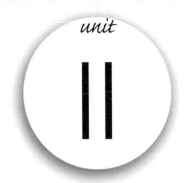

Cellular Function

Chapters 3 to 7

ANATOMY REVIEW
Matching

1. Match each of the following anatomic terms with the appropriate letter in the figure.

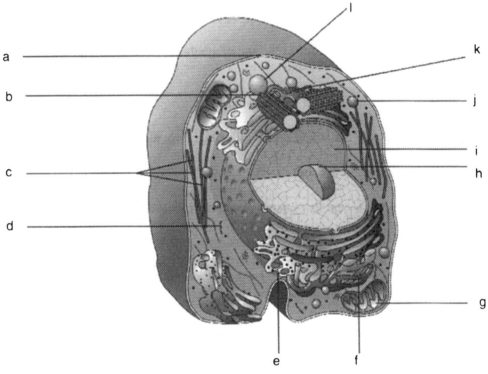

_____	Centrioles	_____	Plasma membrane
_____	Nucleus	_____	Lysosome
_____	Golgi apparatus	_____	Ribosomes
_____	Microtubules	_____	Secretory granule
_____	Rough endoplasmic reticulum	_____	Nucleolus
_____	Mitochondrion	_____	Smooth endoplasmic reticulum

NORMAL ANATOMY AND PHYSIOLOGY REVIEW
True/False

Indicate whether the following statements regarding the anatomy and physiology of cells are true (T) or false (F).

2. _____ The plasma membrane is composed of a lipid bilayer that is highly permeable to water-soluble and charged molecules.

3. _____ Actin and myosin are proteins that are part of the cellular cytoskeleton.

4. _____ The rough endoplasmic reticulum is the site of synthesis of proteins that are destined for secretion from the cell.

5. _____ Glycolysis occurs within the cell's mitochondria.

6. _____ Large quantities of ATP are stored in all cells to provide cellular energy.

7. _____ Glycolysis is an anaerobic process.

8. _____ Oxygen is required to accept low-energy electrons from the mitochondrial electron transport chain enzymes.

9. _____ Channel proteins in the cell membrane allow passive transport of ions.

10. _____ Carrier proteins in the cell membrane are always active transporters.

11. _____ Only cells with voltage-gated ion channels in their plasma membranes are able to conduct action potentials.

12. _____ The RB protein normally functions to bind transcription factors and prevent the cell from initiating its replication cycle.

13. _____ DNA is composed of four nucleotide bases: adenosine, cytosine, uracil, and guanine.

14. _____ Binding of nucleotides is specific such that cytosine (C) always binds with guanine (G).

15. _____ Translation is the process of converting a section of DNA to messenger RNA.

Multiple Choice

Select the one best answer to each of the following questions.

16. Cells differ in structure and function because they:
    A. all have different DNA and genes.
    B. selectively express certain genes that give them their character.
    C. selectively eliminate certain genes from the genome during development.
    D. undergo selective mutations over time.

17. The critical factor for initiation of gene transcription is:
    A. an increase in cellular glucose.
    B. sufficient nutrients.
    C. extracellular signals to initiate the process.
    D. assembly of transcription factors at the promoter area.

18. Which of the following tissues has a limited capacity for replacement of damaged cells?
    A. Epithelium
    B. Smooth muscle
    C. Connective tissue
    D. Nervous tissue

19. The endothelium that lines the blood vessels is categorized as:
    A. connective tissue.
    B. muscle tissue.
    C. nervous tissue.
    D. epithelial tissue.

20. Apoptosis is a physiologic process in which a cell:
    A. divides to form two identical daughter cells.
    B. undergoes purposeful cell suicide.
    C. becomes malignant.
    D. converts to a different cell type.

21. All of the following nucleotide bases are found in RNA except:
    A. adenosine.
    B. cytosine.
    C. thymine.
    D. guanosine.

22. A codon is a:
    A. section of DNA that is spliced out of the original transcript to form messenger RNA.
    B. sequence of nucleotides found on transfer RNA.
    C. gene.
    D. sequence of three nucleotides that code for an amino acid.

23. The lipids that form the cell membrane are amphipathic, meaning that they:
    A. are insoluble.
    B. have both water-soluble and lipid-soluble parts.
    C. evolved from amphibians.
    D. are synthesized from amino acids.

24. The lipid bilayer can form spontaneously in aqueous solution because:
    A. the charge on lipids causes them to attract.
    B. the energy from sunlight is used to move the molecules together.
    C. the lipid bilayer structure allows the water molecules to be less ordered.
    D. the lipid tails form spontaneous covalent bonds.

25. Enzymes function to:
    A. increase the speed of chemical reactions.
    B. determine the direction of chemical reactions.
    C. provide the energy to drive chemical reactions.
    D. make energetically unfavorable reactions occur spontaneously.

PATHOPHYSIOLOGY QUESTIONS
Matching

Match the following genetic abnormalities with their mode of inheritance. Answers may be used more than once.

26. _____ Turner syndrome

27. _____ Klinefelter syndrome

28. _____ Huntington chorea

29. _____ Marfan disease

30. _____ Hemophilia A and B

31. _____ Phenylketonuria

32. _____ Down syndrome

33. _____ Cystic fibrosis

34. _____ Hypertension

A. Autosomal dominant
B. Autosomal recessive
C. X-linked
D. Chromosomal aneuploid
E. Multifactorial

Multiple Choice

Select the one best answer to each of the following questions.

35. Hydropic swelling is a sign of cellular injury associated with:
    A. necrosis.
    B. Na^+-K^+ pump dysfunction.
    C. apoptosis.
    D. aging.

36. Which of the following is not a reversible cellular adaptation?
    A. Atrophy
    B. Hypertrophy
    C. Hyperplasia
    D. Necrosis

37. Glandular tissue normally responds to increased functional demand by:
    A. hypertrophy.
    B. hyperplasia.
    C. metaplasia.
    D. neoplasia.

38. Ischemic death of tissue in visceral organs such as the heart typically produces:
    A. coagulative necrosis.
    B. liquefactive necrosis.
    C. caseous necrosis.
    D. fat necrosis.

39. Cellular injury that results in the production of excessive serum lactate levels is attributable to:
    A. immunologic injury.
    B. nutritional injury.
    C. hypoxic injury.
    D. mechanical injury.

40. Age-related changes in body systems can be described as:
    A. disease processes.
    B. decreased functional reserve.
    C. reversible injury.
    D. compensatory.

41. The normal human genome consists of:
    A. 23 chromosomes.
    B. 22 autosomes and 1 sex chromosome.
    C. 46 chromosomes.
    D. 22 pairs of autosomes.

42. Genes that code for a particular trait come in several forms called:
    A. exons.
    B. introns.
    C. alleles.
    D. phenotypes.

43. Genetic disorders that follow predictable patterns of inheritance are called:
    A. polygenic disorders.
    B. chromosomal aneuploidy.
    C. non-Mendelian disorders.
    D. single-gene disorders.

44. Which of the following chromosomal disorders is categorized as a monosomy?
    A. Klinefelter syndrome
    B. Down syndrome
    C. Turner syndrome
    D. Cri du chat syndrome

45. Characteristics of autosomal dominant disorders include the fact that:
    A. offspring of an affected individual have a 25% chance of being carriers.
    B. offspring of an affected individual have a 25% chance of inheriting the disease.
    C. males are affected more often than females.
    D. unaffected individuals do not transmit the disease.

46. Individuals affected with which genetic disorder are almost always males?
    A. Autosomal dominant disorders
    B. Autosomal recessive disorders
    C. Chromosomal disorders
    D. X-linked disorders

47. The acronym TORCH refers to infectious diseases that may be teratogenic and include all of the following except:
    A. toxoplasmosis.
    B. rubella.
    C. chickenpox.
    D. herpes.

48. The fetus is most vulnerable to teratogenic influences during:
    A. delivery.
    B. conception.
    C. gestational weeks 1 to 3.
    D. gestational weeks 3 to 9.

49. Which of the following would be a significant risk factor for having a fetus with Down syndrome?
    A. Family history of autosomal genetic disorders
    B. Advanced maternal age (>35 years)
    C. Exposure to rubella in the second trimester
    D. Perinatal hypoxemia

50. Proto-oncogene overexpression is associated with the development of:
    A. birth defects.
    B. X-linked genetic defects.
    C. congenital disease.
    D. cancer.

Compare/Contrast

Compare and contrast the features of benign and malignant tumors by filling in the table below.

Characteristic	Benign Tumors	Malignant Tumors
Conventional terminology		
Histology		
Proliferation rate		
Metastasis		
Tumor necrosis		
Recurrence after treatment		
Prognosis		

Multiple Choice

Select the one best answer to each of the following questions.

51. The most important differentiating feature between benign and malignant tumors is:
    A. invasiveness.
    B. a difference in the rate of cell growth within the tumor.
    C. a difference in the tissue of origin.
    D. the size of the tumor.

52. Which of the following tumors is malignant?
    A. Adenoma
    B. Fibroma
    C. Carcinoma
    D. Osteoma

53. Cancer cells exhibit all of the following properties except:
    A. immortality.
    B. excessive proliferation.
    C. nomadic.
    D. high differentiation.

54. Proto-oncogene overactivity increases cellular proliferation through all of the following mechanisms except:
    A. excessive production of growth factors.
    B. excessive production of growth factor receptors.
    C. excessive production of transcription factors.
    D. excessive production of p53.

55. Tumor suppression genes cause cancer when:
    A. they are overproduced in the cell.
    B. they are overactive in the cell.
    C. they are absent from the cell.
    D. they are present in more than one location on the chromosome.

56. Full expression of cancer in a host is a multistep phenomenon. These steps include all of the following except:
    A. initiation.
    B. promotion.
    C. progression.
    D. emigration.

57. Telomerase is an enzyme that:
    A. allows cancer cells to metastasize.
    B. is essential for normal cellular function.
    C. confers immortality to cancer cells.
    D. initiates apoptosis.

58. Tumor "grade" refers to what property of the cancer cells?
    A. Location in the body
    B. Degree of local invasiveness
    C. Extent of metastasis
    D. Histologic characteristics

59. Tumor staging is a process whereby:
    A. the location of tumors in the body is determined.
    B. therapy is initiated and then increased in stages.
    C. tumor cell characteristics are analyzed under the microscope.
    D. the tissue of origin is biochemically determined.

60. If a tumor is characterized according to the TNM system as T2 N1 M0, what is the correct interpretation?
    A. Tumor is localized with no lymph node involvement or metastasis.
    B. Tumor is locally invasive with regional lymph node involvement, no metastasis.
    C. Tumor has spread to distant lymph nodes, no metastasis.
    D. Tumor is disseminated to lymph nodes and distant sites.

Fill in the Blank

61. The energy of the _____ _____ is used by ATP synthase to produce ATP.

62. Cells use _____ receptors to attach to their extracellular matrix.

63. It is estimated that the human genome contains approximately _____ genes.

64. Water always moves passively across cell membranes in response to an _____ gradient.

65. The sodium-potassium ion pump transports _____ sodium ions out of the cell in exchange for two potassium ions.

66. The direction of passive ion flux is determined by the _____ gradient.

67. Protein pores that connect the cell cytoplasm of adjacent cells are called _____ _____.

68. Paracrine signaling occurs when signaling molecules travel through the _____ fluid to target cells, whereas endocrine signaling occurs when signaling molecules travel through the _____.

69. Substitution of one DNA nucleotide for another is called a _____ mutation, whereas loss of one or two nucleotides results in a _____ mutation.

70. Cancer cells arise from tissue _____ cells that are capable of replication.

Case Studies

Sam is a 72-year-old man who is in the clinic with complaints of urinary retention, difficulty initiating the urinary stream, and dribbling. These symptoms are believed by the examining clinician to be associated with an enlarged prostate.

71. A blood sample for prostate specific antigen (PSA) is obtained. PSA is a:
    A. tumor marker for prostate cancer.
    B. histologic examination of the prostate cells.
    C. test for the presence of metastasis.
    D. test for prostate infection (prostatitis).

72. The PSA value is abnormally elevated, and Sam is scheduled for a prostate biopsy procedure. The purpose of the biopsy is to:
    A. obtain tumor cells for histologic examination and grading.
    B. determine whether the tumor cells have invaded locally or metastasized.
    C. stage the tumor.
    D. determine how much of the prostate is cancerous.

73. The results of the biopsy indicate that Sam has "anaplastic cells." This means that:
    A. the tumor cells are benign.
    B. the tumor cells are malignant.
    C. the tumor has already spread to distant sites.
    D. the tumor is well differentiated.

74. Next, Sam is scheduled for a staging procedure to determine the extent of disease. The oncologist notes in the chart that Sam's stage is T1 N0 M0, indicating that:
    A. the tumor has spread beyond the prostate.
    B. there is only regional metastasis.
    C. the tumor is localized within the prostate gland.
    D. the tumor is local and benign.

75. Based on the grading and staging procedures, it is determined that Sam should be treated with surgery to relieve the problem of urinary obstruction, followed by localized irradiation of the prostate gland. Radiation of the prostate will:
    A. selectively kill the tumor cells.
    B. enhance the ability of immune cells to detect and destroy tumor cells.
    C. kill all cells in the irradiated region.
    D. kill the most rapidly dividing cells in the irradiated region.

Sandy is a 36-year-old woman with a strong family history of breast cancer, affecting her mother, sister, and three maternal aunts before the age of 50. Sandy's sister was just diagnosed at age 38, and Sandy is concerned that she may have a genetic predisposition to the disease. A clinical breast examination reveals no significant lumps; however, the breasts are dense and difficult to examine. Sandy is scheduled for a mammography and for genetic testing for *BRCAI* and *BRCAII*.

76. The *BRCAI* and *BRCAII* genes are associated with an inherited form of breast cancer accounting for about 5% of breast cancers. These genes are classified as:
    A. proto-oncogenes.
    B. oncogenes.
    C. tumor suppression genes.
    D. malignancy genes.

77. Sandy's genetic test results indicate that she does not have an abnormality of the *BRCAI* or *BRCAII* genes, but her mammogram reveals a suspicious lesion in the upper outer quadrant of the left breast. Which of the following statements should guide further testing?
    A. Breast cancer is unlikely in view of *BRCA* gene results.
    B. Breast cancer is inevitable in view of family history.
    C. Breast cancer is possible and evaluation of the breast mass is required.
    D. Breast cancer is possible and further genetic testing is advised.

78. Sandy is very upset about the mammography findings and wants further testing to be done immediately. She undergoes a biopsy procedure, the result of which reveals anaplasia of the sample cells. This means:
    A. metastatic breast cancer is present.
    B. benign fibrocystic cells are present.
    C. the breast lesion contains malignant cells.
    D. tumor cells have invaded locally.

79. Sandy is scheduled for surgery to remove the breast lump and evaluate the regional lymph nodes. Her cancer is categorized according to the TNM system as T2 N2 M0 (stage IIIA). This means:
    A. tumor in situ.
    B. several involved regional lymph nodes.
    C. extensive metastasis.
    D. bilateral breast disease.

80. After surgery Sandy is scheduled to receive several rounds of chemotherapy. Chemotherapy is usually administered in cycles because:
    A. cancer cells are in different phases of the cell cycle.
    B. it takes several courses to reach an adequate blood level.
    C. larger doses can be used during each cycle.
    D. cancer cells become more sensitive to the drugs over time.

Mr. and Mrs. Frank are planning to conceive a child and are interested in receiving genetic counseling because of their ages and a history of cystic fibrosis on Mrs. Frank's side of the family. A brief history reveals that Mr. Frank has no known family history of cystic fibrosis or any other genetic disorder. He is 45 years old and has two children from a previous marriage, both of whom are well. Mrs. Frank has a sister with three children, the last of whom was diagnosed with cystic fibrosis. There are no other known family members with this disease. Mrs. Frank is 35 years old and has no children.

81. When assessing the risk for bearing a child with cystic fibrosis, one must consider that the disease is genetically inherited as:
    A. autosomal dominant.
    B. autosomal recessive.
    C. X linked.
    D. chromosomal.

82. Assuming the worst-case scenario that both Mr. and Mrs. Frank have the defective gene for cystic fibrosis, what is the probability of their bearing an affected child?
    A. No risk
    B. 50%
    C. 25%
    D. 75%

83. Mr. and Mrs. Frank decide to undergo genetic testing to determine whether either of them has the cystic fibrosis gene. Mr. Frank does not have it, but Mrs. Frank is heterozygous for the gene (one normal gene, one *CF* gene). With this knowledge one can assess the risk of their bearing a child affected by cystic fibrosis to be closest to:
    A. no risk.
    B. 50%
    C. 25%
    D. 75%

84. Because of their ages, Mr. and Mrs. Frank are concerned about bearing a child with Down syndrome and would like genetic testing to determine their risk prior to initiating the pregnancy. Can this be done?
    A. No, Down syndrome can only be detected after conception.
    B. Yes, Down syndrome risk can be detected by parental blood analysis.

85. After Mrs. Frank becomes pregnant she undergoes amniocentesis to analyze the fetal karyotype. The results indicate that the fetus has two 21st chromosomes. What is the most accurate interpretation of this result?
    A. The child is normal.
    B. Down syndrome is unlikely.
    C. There are no genetic abnormalities.
    D. There are no congenital abnormalities.

ANSWER KEY

ANATOMY REVIEW
Matching

1. b, i, k, c, e, g, a, j, d, l, h, f

NORMAL ANATOMY
AND PHYSIOLOGY REVIEW
True/False

2. F
3. T
4. T
5. F
6. F
7. T
8. T
9. T
10. F
11. T
12. T
13. F
14. T
15. F

Multiple Choice

16. B
17. D
18. D
19. D
20. B
21. C
22. D
23. B
24. C
25. A

PATHOPHYSIOLOGY QUESTIONS
Matching

26. D
27. D
28. A
29. A
30. C
31. B
32. D
33. B
34. E

Multiple Choice

35. B
36. D
37. B
38. A
39. C
40. B
41. C
42. C
43. D
44. C
45. D
46. D
47. C
48. D
49. B
50. D

Compare/Contrast

Characteristic	Benign Tumors	Malignant Tumors
Conventional terminology	Suffix "oma"	Suffix "carcinoma" or "sarcoma"; also leukemia, lymphoma, melanoma
Histology	Similar to tissue of origin, well differentiated	Anaplastic, with abnormal cell sizes and shapes; poorly differentiated
Proliferation rate	Generally slower rate of cycling	Generally more rapid rate of cycling
Metastasis	Never; strictly local	High probability of metastasis
Tumor necrosis	Rare	Common
Recurrence after treatment	Rare	Common
Prognosis	Good	Poor if untreated or detected at late stage

Multiple Choice

51. A
52. C
53. D
54. D
55. C
56. D
57. C
58. D
59. A
60. B

Fill in the Blank

61. proton gradient
62. integrin
63. 30,000
64. osmotic
65. three
66. electrochemical
67. gap junctions
68. interstitial; bloodstream
69. point; frameshift
70. stem

Case Studies

71. A
72. A
73. B
74. C
75. D
76. C
77. C
78. C
79. B
80. A
81. B
82. C
83. A
84. A
85. B

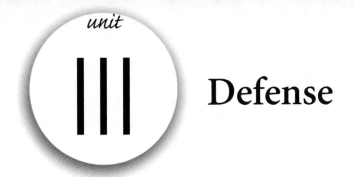
Chapters 8 to 12

ANATOMY REVIEW
Labeling

1. On the diagram below, indicate the blood cell types that evolve from the myeloid and the lymphoid lineages. Include B cells, T cells, red blood cells, platelets, monocytes, and granulocytes (neutrophils, eosinophils, and basophils).

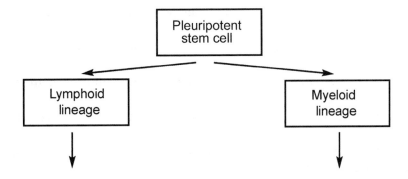

2. On the antibody shown below, indicate the Fab and Fc portions. Label the light and heavy chains. Indicate where the antibody binds its antigen.

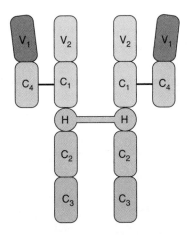

NORMAL ANATOMY AND PHYSIOLOGY REVIEW
True/False

Indicate whether the following statements regarding the anatomy and physiology of the immune system are true (T) or false (F).

3. _____   The primary lymphoid organs are the bone marrow and thymus.

4. _____   The lymphocyte is the most numerous white blood cell (WBC) type in the peripheral blood.

5. _____   The number of neutrophils in the blood increases during acute bacterial infection.

6. _____   Macrophages are mature monocytes.

7. _____   Mast cells are closely related in structure and function to basophils.

8. _____   An increase in neutrophil bands is indicative of acute bacterial infection.

9. _____   T lymphocytes are the principal agents of humoral immunity.

10. _____   Lymphocytes that have CD4 receptors on their cell surface are called T helper cells.

11. _____   B lymphocytes are the principal agents of antibody-mediated immunity.

12. _____   Cytokines are intercellular communication peptides secreted by cells.

13. _____   Previous exposure to foreign antigens is required for activation of neutrophils.

14. _____   Neutrophils marginate along the capillary wall by binding to selectin receptors.

15. _____   Most of the systemic effects of inflammation can be attributed to interleukin-1 (IL-1), IL-6, and tumor necrosis factor α (TNF-α).

16. _____   Cytotoxic T cells bind antigen displayed on cellular major histocompatibility complex (MHC) class II proteins.

17. _____   B cells function as antigen-presenting cells, displaying antigen on their MHC II proteins.

Multiple Choice

Select the one best answer to each of the following questions.

18. All of the following structures are considered secondary lymphoid organs except:
    A. spleen.
    B. tonsils.
    C. bone marrow.
    D. lymph glands.

19. When used in reference to the WBC differential, a "shift to the left" means:
    A. an increase in total WBC count.
    B. an increase in segmented neutrophils.
    C. an increase in neutrophil bands.
    D. an increase in immature lymphocyte blast cells.

20. A normal total WBC count ranges from about:
    A. 4000 to 10,000 cells/μl.
    B. 1500 to 8000 cells/μl.
    C. 10,000 to 15,000 cells/μl.
    D. 500 to 1000 cells/μl.

21. The normal percentage of neutrophils in the WBC count is about:
    A. 20%.
    B. 50%.
    C. 70%.
    D. 90%.

22. The WBCs that migrate to a site of infection quickly are:
    A. monocytes.
    B. lymphocytes.
    C. macrophages.
    D. neutrophils.

23. Basophils and mast cells are unique in that they:
    A. bind and display IgE antibodies on their surfaces.
    B. secrete cytokines.
    C. are nonspecific.
    D. release mediators that enhance inflammation.

24. Macrophages have several roles in the inflammatory and immune response, which include all of the following functions except:
    A. phagocytosis and antigen presentation.
    B. synthesis of serum antibodies.
    C. secretion of inflammatory cytokines.
    D. sentry functions for detection of foreign antigens.

25. Activation of the complement cascade by the classical pathway begins with:
    A. interaction of C3 and foreign antigen.
    B. C1 binding to antigen-antibody complex.
    C. aggregation of C6789 to form the membrane attack complex.
    D. interaction of C1 with foreign antibody.

26. Classic local manifestations of inflammation include all of the following except:
    A. coolness.
    B. redness.
    C. swelling.
    D. pain.

27. When inflammation is chronic, the predominant cell type is:
    A. basophil.
    B. lymphocyte.
    C. neutrophil.
    D. granulocyte.

28. The type of inflammatory exudate characterized as thick, sticky, and high in protein is termed:
    A. serous exudate.
    B. fibrinous exudate.
    C. purulent exudate.
    D. hemorrhagic exudate.

29. Which of the following findings is a systemic sign of inflammation?
    A. Pain
    B. Loss of function
    C. Elevated erythrocyte sedimentation rate ("sed rate")
    D. Swelling

30. The malaise, fever, and increase in acute phase proteins that occur with inflammation are attributed to increases in:
    A. activated complement.
    B. IL-1, IL-6, and TNF-α.
    C. bacterial toxins.
    D. neutrophils.

31. Specific immunity refers to functions of:
    A. natural killer cells.
    B. mononuclear phagocyte system.
    C. mast cells.
    D. B and T lymphocytes.

32. Antigens displayed in association with MHC I complexes on the cell surface are usually:
    A. bacterial in origin.
    B. obtained from intracellular proteins.
    C. obtained by phagocytosis.
    D. bound to antibodies.

33. Lymphocytes that have CD8 proteins on their cell surface are categorized as:
    A. cytotoxic.
    B. helper.
    C. natural killer.
    D. B cells.

34. T helper cells can recognize antigen when:
    A. it is displayed on the cell surface in association with MHC I.
    B. it circulates in the blood or lymph.
    C. it is displayed on the cell surface in association with MHC II.
    D. it is bound to antibody.

35. B cells secrete:
    A. inflammatory cytokines.
    B. complement.
    C. TNF-α.
    D. antibodies.

36. Antibody class is determined by:
    A. the structure of the Fab region.
    B. the structure of the Fc region.
    C. the structure of the B-cell receptor.
    D. the structure of the light chain.

37. The first type of antibody to be secreted upon initial exposure to an antigen is:
    A. IgA.
    B. IgG.
    C. IgE.
    D. IgM.

38. All of the following antibodies circulate as monomers except:
    A. IgD.
    B. IgG.
    C. IgE.
    D. IgM.

39. Plasma cells are:
    A. specialized natural killer cells.
    B. antibody-secreting B lymphocytes.
    C. activated monocytes.
    D. precursors of platelets.

40. Which is an example of passive immunity?
    A. Response to vaccination
    B. Response to disease
    C. Placental transfer of antibodies
    D. Transplant rejection

41. Which of the following immune responses requires T helper cell assistance?
    A. B-cell proliferation and antibody secretion
    B. Activation of the complement cascade
    C. Effective phagocytosis by neutrophils
    D. Macrophage chemotaxis and phagocytosis

42. The antigen-binding specificity of B cells and T cells is determined:
    A. in response to foreign antigen.
    B. randomly, by genetic mechanisms.
    C. by unknown mechanisms.
    D. by antigen-presenting cells.

PATHOPHYSIOLOGY QUESTIONS
Matching

Match the microorganism with its descriptor. Answers may be used more than once or not at all.

43. _____   *Streptococcus pneumoniae*

44. _____   Histoplasmosis

45. _____   Human immunodeficiency virus

46. _____   Scabies

47. _____   Helminths

48. _____   Tinea

49. _____   Epstein-Barr virus

50. _____   *Escherichia coli*

51. _____   *Clostridium botulinum*

52. _____   *Candida*

A. Retrovirus
B. DNA virus
C. Fungus
D. Bacterial rods
E. Bacterial cocci
F. Anaerobe
G. Parasite

Match the disorder on the left with is pathogenetic mechanism on the right. Answers may be used more than once. Some disorders have two answers.

53. _____   Rheumatoid arthritis

54. _____   Asthma

55. _____   Graves disease

56. _____   Hemolytic disease of the newborn

57. _____   Contact dermatitis

58. _____   Poststreptococcal glomerulonephritis

59. _____   Type 1 diabetes mellitus

60. _____   Systemic lupus erythematosus

61. _____   Allergic rhinitis

62. _____   Myasthenia gravis

A. Type I hypersensitivity
B. Type II hypersensitivity
C. Type III hypersensitivity
D. Type IV hypersensitivity
E. Autoimmune disorder

Multiple Choice

Select the one best answer to each of the following questions.

63. Opportunistic infections occur when:
    A. pathogens infect the host.
    B. resident flora cause infectious disease.
    C. bacteria are spread by poor hand washing.
    D. transient bacteria spread among hospitalized patients.

64. Which of the following situations represents a breach in the "first line of defense" against infection?
    A. An abnormally low total WBC count
    B. A "shift to the right" on the WBC differential
    C. Use of an indwelling bladder catheter
    D. Poor nutritional status

65. Certain genotypes have been shown to be associated with a higher risk of developing autoimmune diseases. These genes are of the class:
    A. MHC genes.
    B. T-cell receptor genes.
    C. B-cell antibody genes.
    D. IL genes.

66. Tissue injury associated with autoimmune disease is mediated through:
    A. cytotoxic T cells.
    B. type II and III hypersensitivity responses.
    C. anaphylactic reactions.
    D. type IV hypersensitivity responses.

67. Antibodies are the mediators of all of the hypersensitivity reactions except:
    A. Type I: anaphylactic.
    B. Type II: cytotoxic.
    C. Type III: immune complex.
    D. Type IV: delayed.

68. The antibody type IgE is involved in which type of hypersensitivity reaction?
    A. Type I: anaphylactic
    B. Type II: cytotoxic
    C. Type III: immune complex
    D. Type IV: delayed

69. Graft versus host disease is an example of:
    A. Type I: anaphylactic.
    B. Type II: cytotoxic.
    C. Type III: immune complex.
    D. Type IV: delayed.

70. Severe combined immunodeficiency is a disorder of:
    A. T-cell dysfunction resulting from thymus agenesis.
    B. selective B-cell abnormality.
    C. lymphocyte stem cell failure.
    D. absent WBC growth factors.

71. Chronic stress may cause secondary immunosuppression due to:
    A. overstimulation of the bone marrow leading to failure.
    B. overproduction of cortisol.
    C. impaired antibody production.
    D. excessive catecholamine release.

72. Leukemia is characterized by:
    A. overproduction of blasts in the bone marrow.
    B. overproduction of malignant plasma cells.
    C. the presence of Reed-Sternberg cells.
    D. overproduction of monoclonal antibodies.

73. Generally speaking, the type of leukemia with the best prognosis for cure is:
    A. acute lymphocytic leukemia.
    B. acute myelogenous leukemia.
    C. chronic lymphocytic leukemia.
    D. chronic myelogenous leukemia.

74. The most common cause of death in patients with leukemic disease is:
    A. hemorrhage.
    B. infection.
    C. neurotoxicity from chemotherapeutic agents.
    D. cardiac failure.

75. Manifestations of untreated acute leukemia include all of the following except:
    A. low total WBC count.
    B. low platelet count.
    C. anemia.
    D. bone pain.

76. An important diagnostic feature of chronic myelogenous leukemia is the presence of:
    A. more than 30% blasts in the peripheral blood.
    B. total WBC counts exceeding 75,000 cells/μl.
    C. the Philadelphia chromosome.
    D. infiltration of bony structures.

77. Non-Hodgkin lymphoma is characterized by:
    A. contiguous, predictable pattern of spreading.
    B. the presence of Reed-Sternberg cells on histologic examination.
    C. painless lymph node enlargement.
    D. rare metastasis.

78. Hodgkin disease most commonly presents with:
    A. an enlarged painless cervical lymph node.
    B. an enlarged painless inguinal lymph node.
    C. an elevated total WBC count.
    D. an increase in Reed-Sternberg cells in the peripheral blood.

79. Bence Jones proteins are indicators of:
    A. leukemia.
    B. Hodgkin disease.
    C. non-Hodgkin lymphoma.
    D. plasma cell myeloma.

80. For which of the following diseases is radiation therapy most appropriate?
    A. Acute leukemia
    B. Chronic leukemia
    C. Hodgkin disease
    D. Multiple myeloma

81. Which of the following exposures represents the greatest risk for acquiring human immunodeficiency virus (HIV)?
    A. A blood splash from an HIV-infected individual onto intact skin
    B. Perinatal transmission from an HIV-infected mother to her fetus
    C. Receiving a blood transfusion from a U.S. blood bank
    D. Heterosexual contact using latex condoms

82. HIV virus is called a retrovirus because:
    A. it contains DNA that must be synthesized into RNA to form new virus.
    B. it enters the cell in a reverse fashion through the CD4 receptor.
    C. it contains the enzyme reverse transcriptase.
    D. it reverses the usual sequence of protein synthesis.

83. HIV primarily infects T helper cells and macrophages because:
    A. they have CD4 receptors on their cell surfaces.
    B. other cells do not have the internal machinery to produce new virus.
    C. they are phagocytic and engulf the virus.
    D. the virus knows that these cells must be destroyed to ensure its survival.

84. Some people are resistant to HIV infection because:
    A. they do not have CD4 receptors on their T helper cells.
    B. they lack one or more necessary coreceptors for viral binding and insertion.
    C. their immune systems are stronger.
    D. they were exposed to HIV-like viruses and have developed immunity.

85. Which of the following HIV-positive individuals would appropriately be given the diagnosis of AIDS?
    A. One who developed oral candidiasis
    B. One with a CD4 count of 250 cells/μl
    C. One with *Pneumocystis carinii* pneumonia
    D. One with a herpetic outbreak on the genitalia

86. The HIV virus is known to mutate frequently within an infected individual. This is because:
    A. the virus is trying to escape immune detection.
    B. reverse transcriptase has poor fidelity and makes errors in transcription.
    C. the rate of viral production is so fast that errors in assembly occur.
    D. the selective pressure of antiretroviral drugs increases the mutation rate.

87. Protease inhibitors work by:
   A. blocking the protein binding between glycoprotein (gp) 120 and CD4.
   B. inhibiting reverse transcriptase activity.
   C. inhibiting translation of viral mRNA into protein.
   D. inhibiting protein splicing, viral assembly, and maturation.

Matching

88. Match each letter on the figure below with one of the following terms:

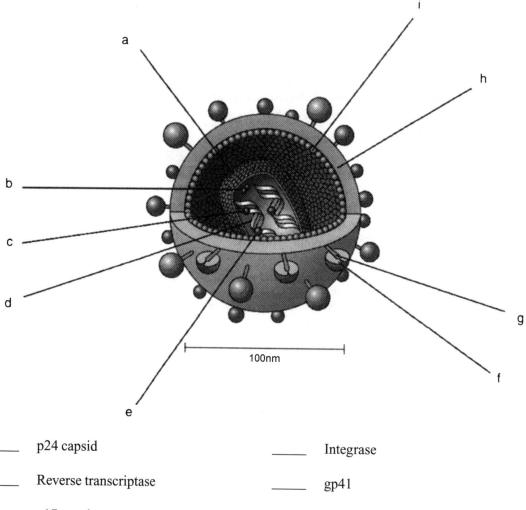

_____ p24 capsid   _____ Integrase

_____ Reverse transcriptase   _____ gp41

_____ p17 matrix   _____ Protease

_____ RNA   _____ gp120

_____ Lipid bilayer

Fill in the Blank

89. Epidemiology is the study of the distribution of disease in a defined _____.

90. The transmission of an infection from one person to another requires five unbroken events in a chain. These are: _____, _____, _____, _____, and _____.

91. An inanimate object such as a contaminated eating utensil that participates in the transmission of infection is called a _____.

92. Certain characteristics increase the risk for contracting an infection and should prompt the nurse to be diligent in prevention and assessment for infection. These include: _____, _____, _____, _____, and _____.

93. When no signs or symptoms of disease are present, the presence of microorganisms on skin and mucous membranes is called _____.

94. The microorganisms that affect humans can be grouped into four broad categories: _____, _____, _____, and _____.

95. Most microorganisms that infect humans remain in the extracellular space; however, _____ must gain entry into cells to establish an infection.

96. Macrophages display numerous receptors on their cell surfaces that help them localize antigens. Some of these receptors bind to opsins, such as the _____ and _____ receptors, whereas others bind directly to microorganisms, including the _____ and _____ receptors.

97. The five classic manifestations of localized inflammation are _____, _____, _____, _____, and _____.

98. The subtype of helper T cell called TH2 releases a cytokine called interleukin-4, which stimulates B cells to produce the _____ type of antibody. Excessive production of this antibody is associated with type I hypersensitivity.

99. Immunodeficiency disorders can be categorized as primary or secondary. Categorize each of the following disorders as primary (P) or secondary (S).
    _____ HIV/AIDS
    _____ Malnutrition
    _____ Cancer
    _____ Severe combined immunodeficiency
    _____ DiGeorge syndrome
    _____ Selective IgA deficiency

100. In some cases a malignant lymphoid cell type presents as lymphoma whereas in other cases it presents as leukemia. The difference between lymphoma and leukemia is considered to be a difference in _____ of the disease.

101. Categorize each of the following hematologic cell malignancies as either myeloid (M) or lymphoid (L):
     _____ Acute monocytic leukemia
     _____ Acute promyelocytic leukemia
     _____ Burkitt lymphoma
     _____ Chronic neutrophilic leukemia
     _____ Polycythemia vera
     _____ Plasma cell myeloma
     _____ Hodgkin disease

102. More than one genotype of HIV virus has been identified; however, the great majority of HIV-infected individuals in the United States, Europe, Australia, and Central Africa have HIV type _____.

103. Three categories of drugs are used to inhibit HIV replication in cells. These are:
     1. _____
     2. _____
     3. _____

104. An HIV-positive individual is diagnosed with AIDS if the CD4$^+$ lymphocyte count falls below _____ cells/µl or if a category C AIDS indicator condition is present.

Case Studies

Ken is a 36-year-old man with a history of IV drug abuse. He was diagnosed as HIV positive 3 years ago and has been taking zidovudine since then. He has generally been well and comes to the clinic for checkups about every 3 months.

105. Ken's lab report today shows that his CD4 lymphocyte count is 198 cells/µl, which is down from his last count 3 months ago. The physician suggests that Ken begin a protease inhibitor medication. The purpose of this medication is to:
     A. block the HIV from entering cells.
     B. prevent the HIV RNA from being transcribed into DNA.
     C. prevent the virus from being transmitted to others.
     D. prevent the release of functional virus from infected cells.

106. Ken agrees to begin the protease inhibitor but wants to stop the zidovudine. Which statement should serve as a basis for response?
     A. Protease inhibitors work better when in combination with a reverse transcriptase inhibitor.
     B. Protease inhibitors must be used in combination or resistance will develop.
     C. Protease inhibitors are a substitute for reverse transcriptase inhibitors.
     D. The protease inhibitor and the reverse transcriptase inhibitor can be alternated.

107. Subsequent testing demonstrates that Ken's viral load is below the level detected by the serum assay. This means that:
     A. he is responding appropriately to therapy.
     B. his protease inhibitor can be discontinued.
     C. his HIV disease has been eliminated.
     D. his reverse transcriptase inhibitor can be discontinued.

108. The finding that Ken's CD4 lymphocyte count is 198 cells/µl means that:
    A. he has less than a year to live.
    B. his diagnosis is changed from HIV disease to AIDS.
    C. he is unlikely to benefit from further therapy.
    D. he is no longer able to mount an immune response.

Jane is a 12-year-old girl with a severe allergy to bee stings. She carries an emergency kit containing epinephrine with her at all times. The last time she was stung she developed wheezing and severe urticaria.

109. Jane's sensitivity to bee stings is an example of:
    A. Type 1 hypersensitivity.
    B. Type 2 hypersensitivity.
    C. Type 3 hypersensitivity.
    D. Type 4 hypersensitivity.

110. Most of the signs and symptoms related to this type of hypersensitivity are attributable to:
    A. activation of complement.
    B. release of inflammatory mediators from mast cells.
    C. excessive production of eosinophils.
    D. production of autoantibodies.

111. The purposes of the epinephrine injection include all of the following except:
    A. stabilizing mast cell membranes.
    B. relaxing bronchial smooth muscle.
    C. supporting arterial blood pressure.
    D. blocking histamine receptors.

112. In addition to avoiding bee stings and immediately treating those that do occur with epinephrine, Jane might benefit from:
    A. immunosuppressive therapy with steroids.
    B. desensitization therapy.
    C. plasmapheresis.
    D. cytotoxic therapy.

Stan is a 58-year-old man in the clinic for evaluation of back pain. He is sent for an x-ray film, which reveals multiple areas of reduced bone density and a compression fracture of the vertebra. His lab work demonstrates an elevated serum calcium level.

113. Which of the following diseases is most consistent with these findings?
    A. Leukemia
    B. Osteoporosis
    C. Plasma cell myeloma
    D. Lymphoma

114. Which of the following findings would help confirm this diagnosis?
    A. Elevated WBC count
    B. Monoclonal antibody spike on electrophoresis
    C. More than 30% blasts in the bone marrow aspirant
    D. Reed-Sternberg cells in biopsy sample

115. Stan undergoes a bone marrow biopsy, the result of which reveals an abnormally high percentage of plasma cells. This means that his disease is a malignancy of:
    A. T cells.
    B. B cells.
    C. granulocytes.
    D. monocytes.

ANSWER KEY

ANATOMY REVIEW
Labeling
1. See textbook Figure 9-2 to check your answer.
2. See textbook Figure 9-31 to check your answer.

NORMAL ANATOMY AND PHYSIOLOGY REVIEW
True/False
3. T
4. F
5. T
6. T
7. T
8. T
9. F
10. T
11. T
12. T
13. F
14. T
15. T
16. F
17. T

Multiple Choice
18. C
19. C
20. A
21. C
22. D
23. A
24. B
25. B
26. A
27. B
28. B
29. C
30. B
31. D
32. B
33. A
34. C
35. D
36. B

37. D
38. D
39. B
40. C
41. A
42. B

PATHOPHYSIOLOGY QUESTIONS
Matching
43. E
44. C
45. A
46. G
47. G
48. C
49. A
50. D
51. F
52. C
53. C, E
54. A
55. B, E
56. B
57. D
58. C
59. B, E
60. C, E
61. A
62. B, E

Multiple Choice
63. B
64. C
65. A
66. B
67. D
68. A
69. D
70. C
71. B
72. A
73. A
74. B
75. A
76. C
77. C
78. A

79. D
80. C
81. B
82. C
83. A
84. B
85. C
86. B
87. D

Matching

88. a, e, i, d, h, c, g, b, f

Fill in the Blank

89. population
90. reservoir, portal of exit, mode of transmission, portal of entry, host susceptibility
91. fomite
92. disrupted skin or mucous membranes, very young or old, immunosuppression, poor nutrition, chronic illness
93. colonization
94. bacteria, fungi, viruses, parasites
95. viruses

96. Fc (IgG); C3b (complement); toll-like; LPS (CD14)
97. redness, warmth, swelling, pain, impaired function
98. IgE
99. P, S, S, P, P, P
100. stage
101. M, M, L, M, M, L, L
102. 1
103. Nucleoside reverse transcriptase inhibitors, nonnucleoside reverse transcriptase inhibitors, protease inhibitors
104. 200

Case Studies

105. D
106. B
107. A
108. B
109. A
110. B
111. D
112. B
113. C
114. B
115. B

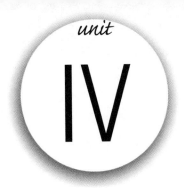
Oxygen Transport, Blood Coagulation, Blood Flow, and Blood Pressure

Chapters 13 to 16

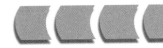

NORMAL ANATOMY AND PHYSIOLOGY REVIEW
Matching

Match the terms in the right column with their definitions in the left column. Not all terms are defined.

Definitions	Terms
1. _____ Not actually cells; fragments of megakaryocytes	A. Oxygen saturation
	B. Bilirubin
2. _____ Cells found in the blood that are important in the inflammatory and immune responses	C. Reticulocyte
	D. Vitamin B_{12}
	E. Hemoglobin
3. _____ A hormone produced by the kidney that is necessary for erythropoiesis	F. pH
	G. Macrophages
	H. Platelets
4. _____ Average volume of blood in the circulatory system of an adult	I. 45%
	J. Partial pressure of O_2
	K. Erythropoietin
5. _____ Major component of red blood cells (RBCs), to which oxygen molecules bind	L. 5 liters
	M. Myeloid stem cell
	N. Monocytes
6. _____ Normal life span of RBCs	O. Metabolic rate
	P. Leukocytes
7. _____ Percentage of the blood that consists of cells	Q. Folate
	R. Lymphoid stem cell
8. _____ Required for adequate synthesis of RBCs; absorbed intestinally in the presence of intrinsic factor	S. Iron
	T. 80 to 120 days
	U. Pleuripotent stem cell
9. _____ Substance released when RBCs break	V. 55%
10. _____ Mature blood cells that leave the bloodstream for the tissues, where they are powerful phagocytes	
11. _____ Bone marrow cell from which all blood cells are derived	
12. _____ Immature RBCs normally representing 1% of the total RBC count	

13. _____ A factor that influences the affinity of hemoglobin for oxygen

14. _____ Factor that, at high levels, stimulates oxygen to bind to hemoglobin

15. _____ Amount of hemoglobin bound to oxygen compared with total amount of hemoglobin in the blood

PATHOPHYSIOLOGY QUESTIONS
Multiple Choice

Select the one best answer to each of the following questions.

16. Which of the following statements about the oxyhemoglobin dissociation curve is true?
    A. The curve shifts to the right with alkalosis.
    B. Hemoglobin levels of below normal will affect the curve.
    C. The curve shifts to the left with an increase in CO_2.
    D. Saturation is most affected when the Pao_2 falls below 60 mm Hg.

17. The pancytopenia associated with aplastic anemia may present with a variety of signs and symptoms including:
    A. bleeding.
    B. increased immune cell function.
    C. increased oxygen saturation levels.
    D. thrombocytosis.

18. Sickle cell crisis causes symptoms related to the anemia and:
    A. vasospasms.
    B. vascular obstruction.
    C. increased risk of acute infection.
    D. bleeding.

19. The most serious hemolytic disease in the newborn occurs because:
    A. the mother has taken medications that cause a decrease in RBC life span.
    B. the mother and father differ in ABO blood type.
    C. Rh factor incompatibility results in antibody formation against fetal RBCs.
    D. maternal RBCs cross the placenta and stimulate antibody production.

20. The earliest clinical indicator of acute blood loss is:
    A. absence of urine production.
    B. tachycardia at rest.
    C. postural hypotension.
    D. cold, clammy skin.

21. Secondary polycythemia would most likely develop in a patient:
    A. who has chronic hypoxemia associated with chronic bronchitis.
    B. who has chronic bleeding associated with a gastric ulcer.
    C. who has dehydration associated with gastrointestinal flu.
    D. who is spending a weekend in the mountains.

22. The arterial oxygen content (CaO_2) for a patient with a PaO_2 of 75 mm Hg, an SaO_2 of 87%, and a hemoglobin level of 12 g/dl would be:
    A. 13.9 ml oxygen/dl.
    B. 1421.5 ml oxygen/dl.
    C. 1399 ml oxygen/dl.
    D. 14.2 ml oxygen/dl.

23. Activation of the intrinsic pathway of coagulation is initiated by:
    A. heparin.
    B. tissue thromboplastin.
    C. blood contact with injured vascular endothelium.
    D. factor X.

24. Fibrinolysis is characterized by:
    A. decreased platelet aggregation.
    B. conversion of plasminogen to plasmin.
    C. conversion of fibrinogen to fibrin.
    D. reduced amounts of fibrin split products.

25. Deficient production of clotting factors would occur if which of the following organs were functioning abnormally?
    A. Liver
    B. Kidneys
    C. Lungs
    D. Bone marrow

26. The proper function of the extrinsic pathway of coagulation is best measured by which of the following laboratory tests?
    A. Prothrombin time (PT)
    B. Activated partial thromboplastin time (aPTT)
    C. Platelet count
    D. Bleeding time

27. A common over-the-counter medication that can alter hemostasis is:
    A. acetaminophen (Tylenol).
    B. antihistamine.
    C. multivitamins.
    D. ibuprofen (nonsteroidal antiinflammatory, NSAID).

28. Vitamin K deficiency in the adult may be due to:
    A. overdosage of heparin.
    B. liver disease.
    C. gallbladder removal.
    D. ingestion of large quantities of green, leafy vegetables.

29. Pathologic activation of the clotting cascade producing widespread coagulation and subsequent bleeding from a deficiency of clotting factors occurs in:
    A. von Willebrand disease.
    B. disseminated intravascular coagulation (DIC).
    C. hemophilia A.
    D. hepatitis.

30. Capillary permeability is greatest in the:
    A. blood-brain barrier.
    B. extremities.
    C. heart.
    D. kidney glomeruli.

31. Flow through a blood vessel is primarily regulated by alteration of its:
    A. length.
    B. wall thickness.
    C. radius.
    D. distending pressure.

32. Blood pressure is highest in the:
    A. capillaries.
    B. pulmonary artery.
    C. vena cava.
    D. aorta.

33. A common cause of edema is:
    A. decreased capillary fluid pressure.
    B. increased interstitial fluid pressure.
    C. decreased interstitial fluid colloid osmotic pressure.
    D. decreased plasma colloid osmotic pressure.

34. Stimulation of the sympathetic nervous system causes constriction of:
    A. bronchioles.
    B. arteries.
    C. capillaries.
    D. lymphatics.

35. Which of the following vessels has the most rapid blood flow (velocity)?
    A. Vena cava
    B. Capillaries
    C. Venules
    D. Arterioles

36. The ability of tissues to maintain local perfusion regardless of systemic arterial pressure is called:
    A. hyperemia.
    B. vascular resistance.
    C. autoregulation.
    D. compensation.

37. Thrombus formation in the arterial system may produce:
    A. ischemia.
    B. thrombophlebitis.
    C. edema.
    D. infection.

38. Risk factors enhancing the development of atherosclerosis include:
    A. increased high-density lipoproteins (HDLs).
    B. high-protein diet.
    C. elevated low-density lipoprotein (LDL) cholesterol levels.
    D. chronic low blood pressure.

39. The "six P's" associated with an acute arterial occlusion include all of the following except:
    A. pallor.
    B. piloerection.
    C. pulselessness.
    D. pain.

40. The most common cause of pulmonary embolism is:
    A. deep vein thrombosis.
    B. varicose veins.
    C. atherosclerosis.
    D. anemia.

41. Mean arterial pressure (MAP) for a patient with a blood pressure of 150/90 would be:
    A. 210 mm Hg.
    B. 80 mm Hg.
    C. 130 mm Hg.
    D. 110 mm Hg.

42. Stimulation of the baroreceptors in the carotid sinus and aortic arch due to increased blood pressure produces:
    A. increased release of norepinephrine.
    B. increased MAP.
    C. increased cardiac output.
    D. increased parasympathetic inhibition of the heart rate.

43. Atrial natriuretic peptide:
    A. is released from the atria in response to decreased preload.
    B. stimulates the release of renin, aldosterone, and antidiuretic hormone.
    C. increases excretion of water and sodium by the kidney.
    D. decreases the glomerular filtration rate.

44. Risk factors for hypertension include:
    A. obesity.
    B. male gender.
    C. white race.
    D. alcohol consumption.

45. A common cause of secondary hypertension is:
    A. anemia.
    B. renal disease.
    C. myocardial infarction.
    D. dissecting aneurysm.

46. The stage of prehypertension is most appropriately managed with:
    A. calcium channel blockers.
    B. β-blockers.
    C. diuretics.
    D. lifestyle modifications.

47. Orthostatic or postural hypotension would be present if a patient has a supine blood pressure (BP) of 118/75 with a heart rate (HR) of 90 and if the following values are obtained when the patient's head is elevated to 90 degrees:
    A. BP 112/85, heart rate 98.
    B. BP 110/80, heart rate 95.
    C. BP 115/70, heart rate 100.
    D. BP 110/75, heart rate 110.

True/False

Indicate whether the following statements are true (T) or false (F).

48. _____ The goal level for antihypertensive therapy in all patients is less than 140/90 mm Hg.

49. _____ Systemic blood vessels are not significantly affected by parasympathetic innervation.

50. _____ Like veins, lymphatic vessels have valves that prevent backflow and enhance forward movement.

51. _____ The major determinant of systemic vascular resistance is the diameter of arterioles.

52. _____ A serious complication of a thromboembolus leaving the right atrium is a cerebrovascular accident (stroke).

53. _____ The greatest risk associated with dissecting aneurysms is rupture.

54. _____ Stimulation of the renin-angiotensin system results in a lowering of MAP.

55. _____ The primary reason blood pressure increases with age is because the heart becomes a less efficient pump.

56. _____ A common cause of lymphedema is removal of lymph nodes with surgery for breast cancer.

57. _____ Blood pressure in the pulmonary vascular bed is higher than that in the systemic vascular bed.

58. _____ *Arteriosclerosis* and *atherosclerosis* are synonymous terms.

59. _____ Systolic blood pressures taken at the dorsalis pedis artery in the foot should be nearly the same as those taken at the brachial artery.

60. _____ The pulse pressure for a patient with a blood pressure of 155/85 mm Hg would be 70.

Fill in the Blank

61. Fill in the anemia table below with E (elevated), N (normal), or D (decreased) for the mean corpuscular volume (MCV) and mean corpuscular hemoglobin concentration (MCHC).

Anemia Disorder	MCV	MCHC
Iron deficiency		
Aplastic		
Vitamin B_{12} deficiency		
Folate deficiency		
Thalassemia		
Hemolytic		
Acute blood loss		
Erythropoietin deficiency		

62. Fill in the hemostasis disorder table below with E (elevated or prolonged), N (normal), or D (decreased) for each laboratory finding.

Hemostasis Disorder	Platelet Count	PT/INR	aPTT	Bleeding Time
Idiopathic thrombocytopenic purpura				
Hemophilia A or B				
Liver disease				
Aspirin use				
DIC				

63. Fill in the blood pressure ranges for each category of blood pressure in the table below using JNC-7 (2003) criteria.

Category	Systolic (mm Hg)	Diastolic (mm Hg)
Normal		
Prehypertension		
Hypertension, stage 1		
Hypertension, stage 2		

64. Mature erythrocytes have no organelles and must rely on _____ for cellular energy production.

65. When red cells are degraded, the porphyrin component of hemoglobin is reduced to _____, which is poorly soluble in water and binds to albumin in the plasma.

66. When fully saturated, each gram of hemoglobin carries approximately _____ ml of oxygen.

67. The normal CaO_2 is about _____ ml of oxygen per deciliter and is calculated by the following formula:

$$CaO_2 = (_____ \times 0.003) + (Hb\ g/dl \times _____ \times _____).$$

68. Under normal conditions about _____ % of the oxygen carried in arterial blood is unloaded at the tissues.

69. The serum erythropoietin level can be helpful in differentiating polycythemia vera from secondary polycythemia because it is elevated in _____ _____ and low in _____ _____.

70. Platelets aggregate together by binding to fibrinogen with their _____ receptors.

71. Aspirin and other NSAIDs inhibit platelet function by inhibiting the enzyme _____, which decreases the production of prostaglandins and thromboxanes.

72. According to Ohm's law (Q = P/R), an increase in resistance (R) will result in a(n) _____ in flow (Q), and an increase in driving pressure (P) will result in a(n) _____ in flow.

73. Driving pressure is calculated by subtracting the pressure at the distal end of a tube (P2) from the pressure at the proximal end (P1). If the MAP is 80 mm Hg and the right atrial pressure (RAP) is 20 mm Hg, then driving pressure through the systemic vessels is _____ mm Hg.

74. An increase in MAP will _____ driving pressure, whereas an increase in RAP will _____ driving pressure.

75. According to Poiseuille's law ($R = 8nl/\pi r^4$), a twofold increase in vessel radius (r) will result in a _____-fold reduction in resistance (R).

76. A twofold increase in vessel length (l) will result in a _____-fold increase in resistance (R).

77. Using the law of Laplace, name three conditions that would increase wall tension: _____, _____, and _____.

78. Calculate the capillary filtration pressure (mm Hg) if capillary hydrostatic pressure is 40 mm Hg, capillary oncotic pressure is 35 mm Hg, tissue hydrostatic pressure is 2 mm Hg, and tissue oncotic pressure is zero: _____.

79. A tissue can increase its rate of blood flow by reducing its _____.

80. According to the American Heart Association, there are specific risk factors for atherosclerosis. List some of the modifiable and nonmodifiable risks below.

Modifiable	Nonmodifiable
1. _____	1. _____
2. _____	2. _____
3. _____	3. _____
4. _____	4. _____
5. _____	5. _____
6. _____	
7. _____	

81. Errors in the measurement of blood pressure have predictable effects. Note the likely effect for each error in the table below:

Error	Effect on Blood Pressure
Blood pressure cuff too large	
Arm positioned above heart	
Arm unsupported	
Less than 1 minute between readings	

82. When assessing blood pressure in children, a reading that is lower than the _____th percentile for age and gender is considered normal.

83. Isolated systolic hypertension is diagnosed when the systolic blood pressure remains above _____ mm Hg but the diastolic pressure remains below _____ mm Hg.

84. When discussing the potential complications of poorly controlled hypertension with a patient, three important organ systems should be mentioned and assessed: _____, _____, and _____.

85. Three categories of antihypertensive medications have been shown to improve outcomes (morbidity, mortality) in patients with hypertension. These are _____, _____, and _____, which are considered to be first-line agents for treatment.

Case Studies

K.T. is a 25-year-old woman who came to the clinic complaining of increasing fatigue during the past few months and a recent onset (this week) of dyspnea and shortness of breath. A diagnosis of anemia is made when her laboratory results indicate a decreased RBC count, decreased hemoglobin, and decreased RBC indices (MCV, MCHC, and MCH).

86. Based on these laboratory values, what type of anemia does K.T. have?
    A. Aplastic anemia
    B. Vitamin B_{12} deficiency anemia
    C. Folate deficiency anemia
    D. Iron deficiency anemia

87. The signs and symptoms of anemia are all related to what common pathophysiologic feature of the condition?
    A. Increased oxygen consumption by tissues
    B. Hypoxemia
    C. Vasodilation
    D. A shift in the oxyhemoglobin dissociation curve

88. A possible cause of K.T.'s anemia is:
    A. bone marrow suppression.
    B. insufficient production of erythropoietin.
    C. autoimmune disease.
    D. chronic excessive blood loss during menstruation.

F.G. is being treated for chronic idiopathic thrombocytopenic purpura.

89. The underlying mechanism of this condition is:
    A. aplastic anemia.
    B. failure of the liver to produce adequate numbers of platelets.
    C. unknown; possibly autoimmune.
    D. aspirin toxicity.

90. F.G., like other patients with this condition, presents with all of the following except:
    A. decreased hemoglobin.
    B. ecchymosis.
    C. petechiae.
    D. hematomas.

91. Laboratory test results indicative of thrombocytopenia, in addition to a low platelet count, would be:
    A. increased PT.
    B. prolonged bleeding time and poor clot retraction.
    C. increased aPTT.
    D. decreased RBC count.

Because S.M. had a heart attack 2 months ago, he and his wife are very motivated to make the necessary lifestyle changes to reduce his risk of having another one. The nurse is working with this couple to reduce his risk factors for atherosclerosis.

92. S.M. is encouraged to raise his HDL levels as a protection against atherosclerosis. The goal for HDL levels should be:
    A. less than 200 mg/dl.
    B. greater than 40 mg/dl.
    C. greater than 160 mg/dl.
    D. flexible; no ideal level has been established.

93. In addition to raising his HDL, S.M. is encouraged to lower his LDL cholesterol by taking medication. The LDL goal for a patient with known coronary heart disease is:
    A. less than 160 mg/dl.
    B. less than 130 mg/dl.
    C. less than 100 mg/dl.
    D. less than 70 mg/dl.

94. Suggested dietary modifications for S.M. should include:
    A. avoidance of hydrogenated and trans fatty acids and oils.
    B. use of only natural fats, such as those from animals and corn oil.
    C. use of sources of simple sugars to substitute for fat calories.
    D. Use of stimulant dietary aids to achieve weight loss.

As part of his routine physical examination, G.H. had his blood pressure checked. It was found to be 170/100 mm Hg. G.H. is 54 years old, is 5 feet 10 inches tall, and weighs 230 pounds. He is a commercial realtor. His serum cholesterol level is 265 mg/dl, his LDL is 170 mg/dl, and his HDL is 24 mg/dl. His father died after a second heart attack, and his mother had a stroke when she was 72; she is now living in a retirement community.

95. G.H. is asked to have his blood pressure measured again to verify that it is still elevated. This is done because:
    A. numerous factors can cause spurious blood pressure elevations.
    B. it is unlikely that his blood pressure is really this high.
    C. everyone experiences "white coat" phenomenon during a physical examination.
    D. no treatment is indicated for a blood pressure of 170/100.

96. In addition to lifestyle modifications, initial drug therapy for hypertension in a patient without specific indicator conditions usually includes:
    A. nitrates.
    B. α_1 receptor antagonists.
    C. calcium channel blockers.
    D. thiazide diuretics.

97. G.H. is not enthusiastic about having treatment for his hypertension. "But I really feel fine," he tells the nurse. The nurse explains that therapy should be initiated now is because:
    A. management of elevated blood pressure now will solve the problem, after which therapy can be stopped.
    B. elevated blood pressure causes organ damage before signs or symptoms are evident.
    C. aggressive management of hypertension will prevent a heart attack or stroke.
    D. if G.H.'s hypertension isn't managed now, it will continue to elevate.

P.R. is 24 years old and 6 months pregnant with her first child. She has had a normal pregnancy to this point, but during this visit her blood pressure is found to have increased from her previous baseline of 116/74 to 150/98. Her nurse practitioner suspects preeclampsia.

98. In addition to hypertension, preeclampsia is characterized by:
    A. nausea and vomiting.
    B. fatigue and lower back pain.
    C. protein in the urine and edema.
    D. retinal changes and rales in the lungs.

99. Three months after delivery of the baby, P.R.'s blood pressure remains elevated at 150/98. A thorough workup reveals no identifiable cause for the high blood pressure, and a diagnosis of _____ is made:
    A. chronic preeclampsia
    B. postpartum hypertension
    C. secondary hypertension
    D. primary or essential hypertension

100. Normally, blood pressure falls slightly during the first 6 months of pregnancy. This is due to:
    A. decreased systemic vascular resistance.
    B. increased cardiac output.
    C. decreased heart rate.
    D. decreased circulating blood volume.

ANSWER KEY

NORMAL ANATOMY AND PHYSIOLOGY REVIEW
Matching

1. H
2. P
3. K
4. L
5. E
6. T
7. I
8. D
9. B
10. G
11. U
12. C
13. F
14. J
15. A

PATHOPHYSIOLOGY QUESTIONS
Multiple Choice

16. D
17. A
18. B
19. C
20. C
21. A
22. D
23. C
24. B
25. A
26. A
27. D
28. B

29. B
30. D
31. C
32. D
33. D
34. B
35. A
36. C
37. A
38. C
39. B
40. A
41. D
42. D
43. C
44. A
45. B
46. D
47. D

True/False

48. F
49. T
50. T
51. T
52. F
53. T
54. F
55. F
56. T
57. F
58. F
59. T
60. T

Fill in the Blank

61.

Anemia Disorder	MCV	MCHC
Iron deficiency	D	D
Aplastic	N	D
Vitamin B_{12} deficiency	E	N
Folate deficiency	E	N
Thalassemia	D	D
Hemolytic	N	N
Acute blood loss	N	N
Erythropoietin deficiency	N	N

62.

Hemostasis Disorder	Platelet Count	PT/INR	aPTT	Bleeding Time
Idiopathic thrombocy-topenic purpura	D	N	N	E
Hemophilia A or B	N	N	E	N or E
Liver disease	N or D	E	N or E	E
Aspirin use	N	N	N	E
DIC	D	E	E	E

63.

Category	Systolic (mm Hg)	Diastolic (mm Hg)
Normal	<120 and	<80
Prehypertension	120-139 or	80-89
Hypertension, stage 1	140-159 or	90-99
Hypertension, stage 2	≥160	≥100

64. glycolysis
65. bilirubin
66. 1.34
67. 20; $Cao_2 = (Pao_2 \times 0.003) + (Hb\ g/dl \times 1.34 \times Sao_2)$.
68. 25
69. secondary polycythemia; polycythemia vera
70. glycoprotein IIb/IIIa
71. cyclooxygenase
72. decrease; increase
73. 60
74. increase, decrease

75. 16
76. two
77. increased distending pressure, increased radius, decreased wall thickness
78. 3
79. resistance
80. *Modifiable:* smoking, hypertension, lipid risks, diabetes, obesity, physical inactivity, hypercoagulable (thrombogenic) state.
Nonmodifiable: age, gender, family history, ethnicity

81.

Error	Effect on Blood Pressure
Blood pressure cuff too large	Falsely low
Arm positioned above heart	Falsely low
Arm unsupported	Falsely high
Less than 1 minute between readings	Falsely high

82. 90
83. 140; 90
84. heart, kidney, brain
85. diuretics, β-blockers, angiotensin-converting
   enzyme inhibitors

Case Studies

86. D
87. B
88. D
89. C

90. A
91. B
92. B
93. C
94. A
95. A
96. D
97. B
98. C
99. D
100. A

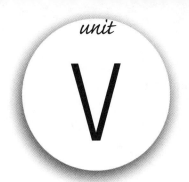

unit

V

Cardiac Function

Chapters 17 to 20

ANATOMY REVIEW
Matching

1. Match each lettered item in the figure with one of the following anatomic terms:

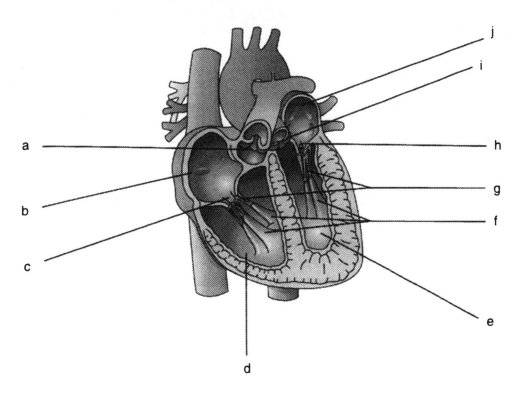

_____ Pulmonary valve	_____ Left atrium
_____ Tricuspid valve	_____ Aortic valve
_____ Right atrium	_____ Mitral valve
_____ Right ventricle	_____ Chordae tendineae
_____ Left ventricle	_____ Papillary muscles

2. Match each lettered item in the figure with one of the following anatomic terms:

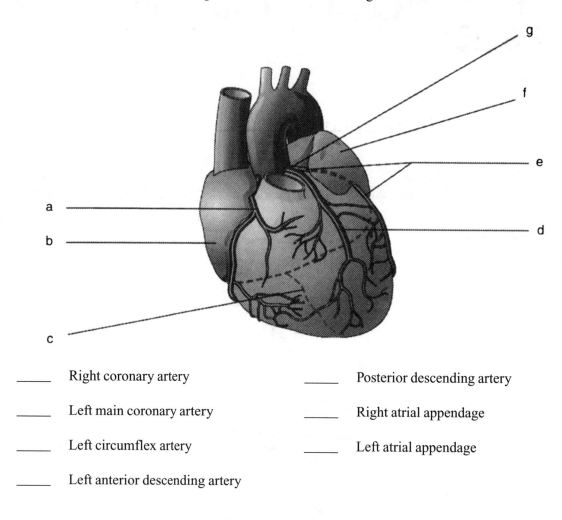

_____ Right coronary artery

_____ Left main coronary artery

_____ Left circumflex artery

_____ Left anterior descending artery

_____ Posterior descending artery

_____ Right atrial appendage

_____ Left atrial appendage

NORMAL ANATOMY AND PHYSIOLOGY REVIEW
True/False

Indicate whether the following statements regarding the anatomy and physiology of the cardiac system are true (T) or false (F).

3. _____ The right atrium and ventricle form the anterior portion of the heart.

4. _____ The point of maximal impulse is normally located at the intersection of the fifth intercostal space and the left midclavicular line.

5. _____ The mitral valve is located between the right atrium and the right ventricle.

6. _____ The pulmonic and aortic valves usually have two cusps (bicuspid).

7. _____ Chordae tendineae tether the aortic and pulmonic valves to the myocardium.

8. _____ Left ventricular muscle is two to three times thicker than right ventricular muscle.

9. _____ The endocardium is the inner surface of the heart chambers.

10. _____ Visceral pericardium is attached to the epicardial surface of the heart.

11. _____ Blood in the pulmonary veins is normally well oxygenated.

12. _____ The left atrium receives blood from the pulmonary artery.

13. _____ The left coronary artery perfuses the posterior aspect of the left ventricle in most people.

14. _____ Normally, the principal determinant of coronary artery resistance is coronary artery radius.

15. _____ The coronary arteries originate in the aorta, just distal to the aortic valve.

16. _____ Most blood flow through the coronary arteries occurs during ventricular systole.

17. _____ The left coronary artery has two principal branches: the left circumflex and the left anterior descending.

Cardiac Cycle Events

18. Label the cardiac cycle events on the figure with the following terms.

A wave   Aortic valve closure

C wave   Aortic valve opening

V wave   Dicrotic notch

Ventricular diastole   Isovolumic contraction

Ventricular ejection   Isovolumic relaxation

Time of S$_1$ Atrial systole

Time of S$_2$

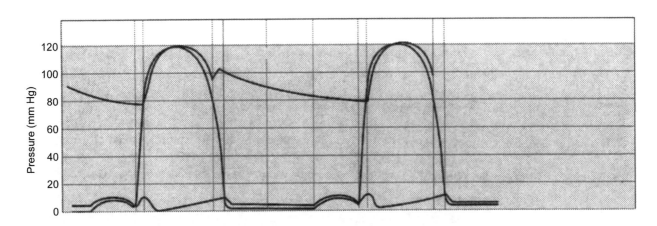

19. Describe the ionic events during each of the five phases of the cardiac action potential.

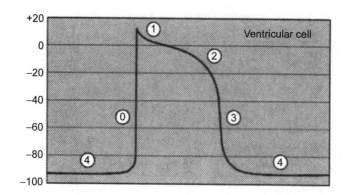

Phase 0:

Phase 1:

Phase 2:

Phase 3:

Phase 4:

Multiple Choice

Select the one best answer to each of the following questions.

20. The myocardial cells of the heart contract synchronously as a syncytium because:
    A. they are connected by gap junctions.
    B. they have one continuous cell membrane.
    C. they are all innervated by the same neuron.
    D. they all have the same rate of spontaneous depolarization.

21. The proteins that make up the contractile apparatus of a myocardial cell include all of the following except:
    A. troponin.
    B. tropomyosin.
    C. actin.
    D. myoglobin.

22. Contraction of cardiac muscle is initiated by:
    A. ATP hydrolysis by myosin head groups.
    B. an increase in free intracellular calcium ion concentration.
    C. opening of voltage-gated potassium channels.
    D. binding of troponin and tropomyosin.

23. The affinity of myosin head groups for binding actin is decreased when myosin binds:
    A. ATP.
    B. GTP.
    C. ADP.
    D. calcium.

24. Relaxation of cardiac muscle is an energy-requiring process because:
    A. energy is required for the sodium-potassium pump.
    B. energy is required to break actin-myosin cross-bridges.
    C. energy is required to pump calcium ions out of the cytosol.
    D. energy is required to close voltage-gated sodium channels.

25. Creatine phosphate:
    A. is a marker of cardiac cell death.
    B. can donate a high-energy phosphate to ADP to form ATP.
    C. is stored in large quantity in most cells.
    D. has different isoforms in different cell types.

26. Which of the following statements about the ventricular myocardial action potential is not correct?
    A. Fast voltage-gated sodium ion channels open during phase 0.
    B. Slow voltage-gated calcium channels are open during phase 2.
    C. Repolarization during phase 3 is accomplished by the sodium-potassium pump.
    D. Voltage-gated potassium channels are open during phases 1, 2, and 3.

27. Pacemaker cells can generate action potentials because:
    A. they are hyperpolarized at rest.
    B. they have receptors for autonomic neurotransmitters.
    C. they spontaneously open cation (Na^+, $Ca2^+$) channels during phase 4.
    D. they spontaneously open chloride channels during phase 4.

28. Sympathetic nervous system action on pacemaker cells:
    A. increases chloride ion conductance.
    B. increases potassium ion efflux.
    C. decreases sodium ion influx.
    D. increases sodium ion conductance.

29. Parasympathetic nervous system action on pacemaker cells:
    A. increases calcium ion conductance.
    B. increases potassium ion efflux.
    C. increases sodium ion conductance.
    D. decreases calcium ion conductance.

30. The usual sequence of depolarization of the ventricles begins with:
    A. right ventricular muscle.
    B. septal muscle.
    C. left ventricular apex muscle.
    D. lateral wall of left ventricle.

31. The PR interval of the electrocardiogram (ECG) corresponds to depolarization of:
    A. the atria.
    B. the AV node.
    C. the atria, AV node, and His-Purkinje fibers.
    D. the ventricular septum.

32. Cardiac output is the product of heart rate and:
    A. contractility.
    B. blood pressure.
    C. stroke volume.
    D. preload.

33. Which of the following would result in a decrease in cardiac output?
    A. Increased preload
    B. Increased contractility
    C. Increased afterload
    D. Increased heart rate

34. Contractility is enhanced by factors that increase:
    A. preload.
    B. stroke volume.
    C. baroreceptor activity.
    D. intracellular free calcium ions.

35. The Frank-Starling law of the heart suggests that increased preload will:
    A. decrease cardiac workload.
    B. increase cardiac heart rate.
    C. increase stroke volume.
    D. increase afterload.

PATHOPHYSIOLOGY QUESTIONS
Compare/Contrast

36. Compare and contrast myocardial infarction (MI) and stable angina by filling in the table.

Characteristic	MI	Stable Angina Pectoris
Pain character		
Electrocardiographic findings		
Serum marker elevations		

Multiple Choice

Select the one best answer to each of the following questions.

37. The most common cause of cardiac ischemia is:
   A. hypoxemia.
   B. excessive myocardial oxygen demand.
   C. anemia.
   D. reduced coronary artery blood flow.

38. Ischemic heart disease is nearly always a consequence of:
   A. atherosclerosis.
   B. dysrhythmias.
   C. primary cardiomyopathies.
   D. carditis.

39. Which of the following coronary lesions is thought to be the first symptomatic type?
   A. Type I
   B. Type II
   C. Type III
   D. Type IV

40. Chronic partial occlusion of a coronary artery is associated with the clinical syndrome of:
   A. unstable angina.
   B. stable angina.
   C. MI.
   D. rest angina.

41. The clinical syndromes of coronary heart disease include all of the following except:
   A. stable angina pectoris.
   B. MI.
   C. chronic ischemic cardiomyopathy.
   D. myocarditis.

42. Stable angina pectoris:
   A. results in permanent myocardial cell damage.
   B. is detected by elevated serum marker proteins.
   C. is usually relieved by rest.
   D. rarely lasts longer than 30 seconds.

43. Which of the following is considered the least specific serum indicator of myocardial cell death?
   A. Myoglobin
   B. Troponin I
   C. Creatine kinase, myocardial bound (CK-MB)
   D. Troponin T

44. Acute cardiac ischemia is indicated on the ECG by:
   A. abnormally large Q waves.
   B. abnormally small R waves.
   C. ST-segment elevation.
   D. inverted P waves.

45. The compensatory responses that are triggered following MI serve to:
    A. protect the heart from damage.
    B. maintain cardiac output.
    C. reduce myocardial oxygen consumption.
    D. reduce cardiac workload.

46. The objectives of treatment for acute coronary syndrome are to improve coronary perfusion and to:
    A. reduce myocardial oxygen demand.
    B. reverse the atherosclerotic process.
    C. remove all potential risk factors.
    D. begin antilipid therapy.

47. Stenosis of a cardiac valve results in:
    A. a back flow of blood through the valve.
    B. extra "volume" work for the heart.
    C. a pressure gradient across the valve when open.
    D. a bounding pulse.

48. The murmur of aortic stenosis:
    A. occurs during ventricular diastole.
    B. is heard best at the apex.
    C. radiates to the neck.
    D. obliterates S_1 and S_2.

49. Mitral regurgitation:
    A. results in large left atrial V waves on the atrial pressure monitor.
    B. produces a diastolic murmur.
    C. increases left ventricular afterload.
    D. produces a pressure gradient across the mitral valve during diastole.

50. Bacterial endocarditis most commonly affects valves:
    A. on the left side of the heart.
    B. that are structurally abnormal.
    C. of elderly individuals.
    D. of patients with ischemic cardiomyopathy.

51. Myocarditis is an inflammatory disorder that:
    A. is most commonly associated with streptococcal infections.
    B. often leads to dilated cardiomyopathy.
    C. results in hypertrophy of all four chambers of the heart.
    D. impairs left ventricular filling.

52. Cardiac tamponade compresses the heart chambers and produces:
    A. arterial hypertension.
    B. accentuated heart sounds.
    C. adventitious heart sounds (S_3, S_4).
    D. pulsus paradoxus.

53. Which of the following findings is most indicative of pericarditis?
   A. Chest pain
   B. Pericardial friction rub
   C. Bounding pulse
   D. Displaced point of maximal impulse

54. Acyanotic congenital heart defects include:
   A. tetralogy of Fallot.
   B. transposition of the great vessels.
   C. truncus arteriosus.
   D. patent ductus arteriosus.

55. Congenital heart defects that produce left-to-right shunts:
   A. cause systemic hypoxemia.
   B. increase right ventricular workload.
   C. are cyanotic lesions.
   D. are without consequence.

56. Heart failure has occurred when:
   A. cardiac output falls below 5 L/min.
   B. MI destroys more than 20% of the heart muscle.
   C. high workload is imposed on the heart.
   D. cardiac output is insufficient to meet the needs of the body.

57. The most common cause of heart failure is:
   A. hypertension.
   B. coronary heart disease.
   C. hypertrophic cardiomyopathy.
   D. valvular dysfunction.

58. Patients with diastolic heart failure have symptoms of congestive heart failure, but:
   A. the cardiac output is normal.
   B. the ejection fraction is greater than 0.50.
   C. there is no edema formation.
   D. they are volume depleted.

59. Left-sided heart failure is characterized by:
   A. pulmonary congestion.
   B. jugular vein distention.
   C. dependent edema in the legs.
   D. bounding pulses.

60. Left-sided heart failure may lead to right-sided heart failure owing to:
   A. excessive volume retention.
   B. poor perfusion of the right coronary artery.
   C. increased right ventricular afterload.
   D. arterial hypotension.

61. Most patients with CHF need medications to:
    A. reduce afterload.
    B. increase contractility.
    C. reduce preload.
    D. reduce heart rate.

62. Although the best treatment for patients with diastolic heart failure is unknown, some drugs are thought to be contraindicated, including:
    A. diuretics.
    B. β-blockers.
    C. Angiotensin-converting enzyme (ACE) inhibitors.
    D. inotropic agents.

63. Which of the following agents have been shown to reduce mortality in patients with systolic heart failure?
    A. Loop diuretics
    B. Inotropic agents (β agonists, digitalis)
    C. ACE inhibitors and β-blockers
    D. Calcium channel blockers

64. All of the following are characteristics of normal sinus rhythm except:
    A. PR interval 0.12 to 0.20 second.
    B. one P wave for each QRS complex.
    C. rate of 60 to 100 beats/min.
    D. QRS duration of 0.4 to 1.0 second.

65. Which of the following dysrhythmias is attributed to reentry mechanism?
    A. Ventricular fibrillation
    B. Asystole
    C. Sinus bradycardia
    D. Junctional escape rhythm

66. A first-degree conduction block is characterized by:
    A. bradycardia.
    B. dropped P waves.
    C. prolonged PR interval.
    D. widened QRS.

67. Type 1 (Wenckebach) second-degree block is characterized by:
    A. dropped P waves with consistent PR interval.
    B. no apparent association between P waves and QRS complexes.
    C. progressive lengthening of PR interval until a P wave is not conducted.
    D. bizarre-looking QRS complexes.

68. The most important consideration in determining treatment for dysrhythmias is:
    A. how frequently they occur.
    B. whether they are causing symptoms.
    C. the underlying disease process.
    D. how bizarre the complexes appear.

69. The common finding in all types of circulatory shock is:
    A. low blood volume.
    B. low cardiac output.
    C. poor prognosis.
    D. cellular hypoxia.

70. In the early, compensated stage of circulatory shock, blood pressure is maintained owing to:
    A. increased cardiac output.
    B. increased systemic vascular resistance.
    C. increased preload.
    D. venoconstriction.

71. An increased serum lactate level (lactic acidosis) is commonly used as a marker of:
    A. cell death.
    B. anaerobic metabolism.
    C. inflammation.
    D. early shock.

72. A reduced oxygen extraction rate as indicated by a high systemic venous oxygen saturation is associated with:
    A. cardiogenic shock.
    B. hypovolemic shock.
    C. neurogenic shock.
    D. septic shock.

73. Types of shock categorized by abnormal distribution of cardiac output (distributive shock) include all of the following except:
    A. hypovolemic shock.
    B. septic shock.
    C. anaphylactic shock.
    D. neurogenic shock.

74. Septic shock is characterized by an abnormally low systemic vascular resistance owing to:
    A. high cardiac output.
    B. cytokine-induced production of nitric oxide.
    C. sympathetic nervous system dysfunction.
    D. widespread release of histamine.

Fill in the Blank

75. Three important characteristics of vulnerable coronary plaques are exposure to high shear stress, _____, and _____.

76. Five syndromes of coronary heart disease can be differentiated. These include two chronic presentations, _____ and _____, and three acute presentations, _____, _____, and _____. In practice MI and unstable angina are similar at the onset, and the term _____ is applied to both.

77. The risk of sustaining a coronary event is higher in those with elevated high-sensitivity C-reactive protein levels, indicating that _____ is an important etiologic factor for coronary heart disease.

78. A patient who presents at the emergency department with chest pain and ST elevation on the ECG is a candidate for _____ therapy.

79. A patient who presents at the emergency department with acute coronary syndrome and ST elevation that progresses to MI is diagnosed with ST elevation myocardial infarction (STEMI), whereas a similar patient whose ST elevation does not progress to MI is diagnosed with _____ _____.

80. A patient who does not have ST elevation on the ECG but still suffers an acute MI as evidenced by elevated serum cardiac enzymes is diagnosed with _____.

81. A person who is exhibiting signs and symptoms of acute coronary syndrome should be directed to take a(n) _____ orally immediately.

82. Rheumatic heart disease and rheumatic fever are uncommon but severe consequences of infection with _____.

83. Individuals who experience rheumatic fever have a _____ % chance of recurrence if they are reinfected and should receive chronic prophylactic antibiotic therapy.

84. In North America, most cases of myocarditis are thought to be a consequence of _____ infections; however, the infective organism is rarely identified.

85. Defects in the structure of myocardial _____ proteins are thought to cause most forms of hypertrophic cardiomyopathy.

Case Studies

P.J. is a 67-year-old man with a long history of stable angina who is treated with nitroglycerin tablets as needed for chest pain. He has mild hypertension, which is well controlled by diet and an ACE inhibitor.

86. P.J. has noticed that his chest pain is occurring with increasing frequency, and less activity is required to initiate the symptoms; however, the pain subsides quickly with rest and one or two nitroglycerin tablets. These symptoms are consistent with a diagnosis of:
A. stable angina.
B. progressive angina.
C. unstable angina.
D. variant angina.

87. P.J. should be counseled to seek medical care immediately when:
A. chest pain occurs more than three to five times per week.
B. mild shortness of breath accompanies the chest pain.
C. chest pain is not relieved within 5 minutes.
D. chest pain occurs at rest or is not relieved within 15 minutes.

88. Effective control of P.J.'s blood pressure is important for all of the following reasons except:
A. high blood pressure is a risk factor for atherosclerosis.
B. high blood pressure increases left ventricular afterload.
C. high blood pressure reduces coronary artery perfusion pressure.
D. high blood pressure contributes to development of left ventricular hypertrophy.

89. One morning at about 4:00 AM. P.J. is awakened from sleep with chest pain and shortness of breath. The pain is much more severe than his usual anginal pain and radiates to the jaw and left arm. He is diaphoretic and pale. His wife calls for emergency assistance, and P.J. is transported to the local emergency department. Upon admission the ECG shows significant ST-segment elevation, which indicates:
    A. acute coronary syndrome.
    B. impending dysrhythmia.
    C. recent MI.
    D. cardiac irritation.

90. The ST elevation is noted only in leads II, III, and aVF, indicating that the affected area of the heart is the:
    A. right ventricle.
    B. intraventricular septum.
    C. anterior wall of the left ventricle.
    D. inferior wall of the left ventricle.

91. It is decided that P.J. should receive a tissue plasminogen activator (tPA). This agent is used because:
    A. acute ischemia is usually caused by a thrombus in the coronary artery.
    B. it reverses the atherosclerotic process in the coronary arteries.
    C. it decreases myocardial oxygen consumption.
    D. it relaxes smooth muscle and prevents coronary vasospasm.

92. At the time of admission a blood sample is taken to determine whether P.J. has suffered an MI. Which of the following laboratory findings would indicate MI?
    A. Elevated creatine phosphate
    B. Elevated total creatine kinase
    C. Elevated troponin I
    D. Elevated erythrocyte sedimentation rate

93. While P.J. is recovering from his cardiac event he is monitored by continuous electrocardiography. On the day after hospital admission he is noted to have a heart rate of 64 beats/min and a PR interval of 0.22 second. The QRS is normal, and there is one P wave for each QRS. This rhythm is termed:
    A. sinus bradycardia.
    B. normal sinus rhythm.
    C. first-degree heart block.
    D. sinus arrhythmia.

94. P.J. is tolerating the rhythm well with no symptoms. Which of the following would be an appropriate action to take at this time?
    A. Prepare to insert a pacemaker
    B. Administer atropine
    C. Do nothing; this is a normal rhythm
    D. Continue monitoring and assessing for symptoms

95. Despite his treatment, P.J. develops pathologic Q waves on his ECG. Based on this finding, he is diagnosed with:
    A. unstable angina.
    B. critical coronary stenosis.
    C. MI.
    D. persistent coronary vasospasm.

K.C. is an 86-year-old woman in generally good health who presents to the clinic with complaints of increasing shortness of breath and reduced activity tolerance. She has no significant cardiac history. Her blood pressure is 110/60, heart rate is 92 beats/min. There is a grade IV systolic murmur that radiates to the neck.

96. Considering K.C.'s age and the nature of the cardiac murmur, this is most likely:
    A. mitral stenosis.
    B. mitral regurgitation.
    C. aortic stenosis.
    D. aortic regurgitation.

97. Auscultation of K.C.'s chest reveals bilateral fine crackles in the bases bilaterally, indicating:
    A. right-sided heart failure.
    B. left-sided heart failure.
    C. pneumonia.
    D. acute respiratory distress syndrome.

98. K.C. is scheduled for surgical valve replacement and recovers well. Her ejection fraction after surgery is about 0.40. Ejection fraction is calculated:
    A. the same as stroke volume.
    B. as the stroke volume divided by the end diastolic volume.
    C. as stroke volume × heart rate.
    D. as cardiac output × vascular resistance.

99. An ejection fraction of 0.40 indicates:
    A. mild systolic dysfunction.
    B. mild diastolic dysfunction.
    C. moderate diastolic dysfunction.
    D. no significant left ventricular dysfunction.

100. K.C. is discharged on an ACE inhibitor medication. All of the following are expected effects of ACE inhibitors except:
    A. preload reduction.
    B. increased contractility.
    C. reduced systemic vascular resistance.
    D. inhibition of left ventricular hypertrophy.

K.K. is a 20-year-old man who was completely healthy until he collapsed during a collegiate basketball game. He was resuscitated on the court and transported to the hospital.

101. Evaluation of K.K.'s 12-lead ECG reveals significant left ventricular hypertrophy, but no evidence of ischemia. His heart rate is 60 beats/min and his blood pressure is 116/70. Considering these findings and the above scenario, K.K. should be evaluated for:
    A. coronary heart disease.
    B. hypertensive heart disease.
    C. hypertrophic cardiomyopathy.
    D. myocarditis.

102. K.K.'s echocardiogram demonstrates extreme septal hypertrophy, and so his collapse on the basketball court is attributed to:
    A. acute MI.
    B. abnormal ventricular conduction pathway.
    C. acute myocardial regurgitation.
    D. acute aortic outflow obstruction.

103. The decision is made to perform surgery to resect a portion of the septum. Postoperatively K.K.'s ECG demonstrates frequent nonconducted P waves (dropped beats) with a consistent PR interval for conducted beats and a wide QRS. This rhythm is called:
    A. first-degree block.
    B. second-degree block, Mobitz type 1 (Wenkebach).
    C. second-degree block, Mobitz type 2.
    D. third-degree block.

104. Which of the following is the most appropriate response to K.K.'s rhythm disturbance?
    A. Monitor only; this rhythm rarely progresses.
    B. Prepare to initiate ventricular pacing if the block is symptomatic or progresses.
    C. Initiate antidysrhythmic medications.
    D. Administer atropine to increase the heart rate.

105. K.K.'s family should be advised that his disorder:
    A. is genetic and family members should be evaluated.
    B. requires absolute activity restriction.
    C. is cured by surgery and no further therapy is necessary.
    D. will progress to heart failure within a few years.

ANATOMY REVIEW
Matching

1. a, c, b, d, e, j, i, h, g, f
2. a, g, e, d, c, b, f

NORMAL ANATOMY AND PHYSIOLOGY REVIEW
True/False

3. T
4. T
5. F
6. F
7. F
8. T
9. T
10. T
11. T
12. F
13. F
14. T
15. T
16. F
17. T

Cardiac Cycle Events

18. See Figure 17-6 in textbook.

19. Phase 0: influx of Na^+ through fast sodium channels
    Phase 1: cessation of Na^+ influx, beginning of K^+ efflux
    Phase 2: influx of Ca^{2+} through slow calcium channel and continued but slower K^+ efflux
    Phase 3: closure of calcium channels, rapid K^+ efflux
    Phase 4: rest, minimal ionic flux

Multiple Choice

20. A
21. D
22. B
23. A
24. C
25. B
26. C
27. C
28. D
29. B
30. B
31. C
32. C
33. C
34. D
35. C

PATHOPHYSIOLOGY QUESTIONS
Compare/Contrast

36.

Characteristic	MI	Stable Angina Pectoris
Pain character	Severe, crushing, substernal may radiate to jaw, neck, left arm. May have nausea diaphoresis, impending doom, shortness of breath. May occur at rest or with activity. Lasts more than 15 minutes despite rest, nitroglycerin	Predictable onset with activity, relieved by rest. Usually lasts less than 5 minutes
Electrocardiographic findings	Acute: ST elevation, T wave inversions Evolved: Large Q waves	May be none. May have transient ST changes during pain
Serum marker elevations	Elevated myoglobin, troponins I and T, CK-MB	No elevations

Multiple Choice

37. D
38. A
39. D
40. B
41. D
42. C
43. A
44. C
45. B
46. A
47. C
48. C
49. A
50. B
51. B
52. D
53. B
54. D
55. B
56. D
57. B
58. B
59. A
60. C
61. C
62. D
63. C
64. D
65. A
66. C
67. C
68. B
69. D
70. B
71. B
72. D
73. A
74. B

Fill in the Blank

75. large lipid core; thin cap
76. stable angina, ischemic cardiomyopathy, unstable angina, MI, sudden cardiac death, acute coronary syndrome
77. inflammation
78. thrombolytic
79. unstable angina
80. NSTEMI (non-ST elevation MI)
81. aspirin
82. Group A β-hemolytic streptococci
83. 50
84. viral
85. cytoskeletal or sarcomere

Case Studies

86. A
87. D
88. C
89. A
90. D
91. A
92. C
93. C
94. D
95. C
96. C
97. B
98. B
99. A
100. B
101. C
102. D
103. C
104. B
105. A

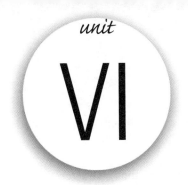

unit

VI

Respiratory Function

Chapters 21 to 23

ANATOMY REVIEW
Matching

1. Match each lettered item in the figure with one of the following anatomic terms:

_____ Alveoli

_____ Nasal cavity

_____ Bronchi

_____ Esophagus

_____ Right lung of patient

_____ Laryngopharynx

_____ Nasopharynx

_____ Bronchioles

_____ Oropharynx

_____ Trachea

_____ Left lung of patient

NORMAL ANATOMY AND PHYSIOLOGY REVIEW
True/False

Indicate whether the following statements regarding the anatomy and physiology of the respiratory system are true (T) or false (F).

2. _____ The larynx is anatomically part of the lower airway but performs functions characteristic of the upper airway.

3. _____ Cilia are located throughout the airway and are responsible for the production of mucus.

4. _____ Aspiration of food into the airway is prevented by closure of the trachea with swallowing.

5. _____ The carina is the anatomic end of the trachea, where the two mainstem bronchi originate.

6. _____ Aspirated materials tend to go into the right mainstem bronchus because it is shorter, wider, and at less of an angle from the trachea.

7. _____ The right lung has two lobes whereas the left has three.

8. _____ Surfactant is produced by the columnar epithelial cells lining the airways.

9. _____ Stimulation of the sympathetic branch of the autonomic nervous system results in the release of acetylcholine, which causes constriction of smooth muscle in the bronchi and bronchioles.

10. _____ Cough reflex receptors are located at the epiglottis and carina.

11. _____ Gas exchange occurs between the alveoli and capillaries (alveolar unit) by the physical process of diffusion.

12. _____ A reduction in the number of alveoli is to be expected as a part of the aging process.

13. _____ Blood is delivered to the lungs by the pulmonary vein, and oxygenated blood leaves the lungs via the pulmonary artery.

14. _____ Expiration is a passive process, primarily due to the elastic recoil of the lung tissue.

15. _____ An increase in lung compliance is associated with aging.

16. _____ The chemoreceptor center in the medulla is stimulated primarily by an increase in arterial CO_2.

PATHOPHYSIOLOGY QUESTIONS
Compare/Contrast

Compare and contrast chronic bronchitis and emphysema by filling in the following table. Write "yes" or "no" in the appropriate column.

Characteristic	Chronic Bronchitis	Emphysema
Early hypoxemia		
Early CO_2 retention		
Productive cough		
Increased A-P diameter		
Cor pulmonale		

Multiple Choice

Select the one best answer to each of the following questions.

17. Bronchiolitis, commonly seen in infants due to respiratory syncytial virus, is characterized by:
    A. airway inflammation and mucus formation.
    B. atrophy of smooth muscle of the airway.
    C. increased compliance of lung tissue.
    D. thin secretions from the nose.

18. Which of the following statements regarding cystic fibrosis is correct?
    A. It is caused by a bacterial infection.
    B. It can be prevented by a vaccine.
    C. It is associated with a genetic defect in chloride ion transport.
    D. It affects only the pulmonary system.

19. Signs or symptoms of tracheobronchial obstruction include all of the following except:
    A. stridor.
    B. wheezing.
    C. sternal retractions.
    D. crackles.

20. A classic clinical finding when a patient has epiglottitis is:
    A. pain and difficulty swallowing.
    B. pain with inspiration.
    C. unequal thoracic expansion.
    D. earaches.

21. Croup is a syndrome, a collection of signs and symptoms that may be due to several etiologic factors. The most characteristic finding in croup is:
    A. earaches.
    B. barking cough with respiratory stridor.
    C. enlarged lymph nodes in the neck.
    D. marked fever.

22. An abnormal opening between the esophagus and trachea is called:
    A. an atresia.
    B. a fistula.
    C. atelectasis.
    D. a perforation.

23. Extrinsic asthma:
    A. is mediated by IgG.
    B. presents with different signs and symptoms than intrinsic asthma.
    C. is due to an antigen-antibody reaction on IgE-bearing mast cells.
    D. often is precipitated by exercise.

24. Air trapping associated with chronic obstructive diseases results in an increase in which of the following components of pulmonary function testing?
    A. Residual volume
    B. Forced expiratory volume in one second (FEV_1)
    C. Vital capacity
    D. Expiratory reserve volume

25. Acute and chronic bronchitis differ in which of the following ways?
    A. Chronic bronchitis is caused by repeated infections.
    B. Acute bronchitis is not associated with increased mucus production.
    C. Acute bronchitis produces arterial blood gas changes reflecting significant hypoxemia.
    D. Chronic bronchitis results in airway changes that are irreversible.

26. High-dose oxygen therapy must be used cautiously in patients with chronic bronchitis because:
    A. V/Q changes can result in further elevations in partial pressure of carbon dioxide in arterial blood ($Paco_2$).
    B. pulmonary vasoconstriction will worsen, increasing the work of the right heart.
    C. respiratory smooth muscle constriction will result in increased air trapping.
    D. peripheral chemoreceptors will be depressed and the patient will stop breathing.

27. Which of the following assessment findings is indicative of an asthma attack?
    A. Wheezing
    B. Thin, watery mucus production
    C. Nonproductive cough
    D. Fever

28. Pathophysiologic differences between emphysema and chronic bronchitis include the fact that:
    A. emphysema is characterized by hypersecretion of goblet and mucus cells.
    B. chronic bronchitis commonly results in polycythemia to compensate for persistent hypoxemia.
    C. chronic bronchitis produces destruction of alveolar walls.
    D. emphysema is due to chronic inflammation resulting in fibrotic airways.

29. Arterial blood gases for a patient with mild to moderate emphysema would reflect:
    A. Severe hypoxemia.
    B. increased $Paco_2$.
    C. near-normal Pao_2 and normal to low $Paco_2$.
    D. respiratory failure.

30. Pursed-lip breathing is commonly used by patients with emphysema because it:
    A. increases the pressure gradient for gas exchange.
    B. helps strengthen accessory respiratory muscles.
    C. decreases small airway collapse during expiration.
    D. prolongs inspiration to allow gas to reach distal air sacs.

31. Restrictive pulmonary diseases are associated with which of the following pulmonary function test results?
    A. Increased total lung capacity
    B. Increased residual volume
    C. Increased functional residual capacity
    D. Decreased vital capacity

32. Occupational lung diseases such as pneumoconiosis:
    A. result from chronic inhalation of particles of inert materials.
    B. are characterized by early marked elevations in Pa_{CO_2}.
    C. produce an increase in lung compliance.
    D. are due to antigen-antibody reactions.

33. The pathology of acute respiratory distress syndrome produces hypoxemia that is refractory to oxygen therapy. This is because of:
    A. decreased pulmonary compliance.
    B. increased functional residual capacity.
    C. profound intrapulmonary shunting past alveoli with no ventilation.
    D. significant dyspnea.

34. The underlying pathologic condition of infant respiratory distress syndrome (hyaline membrane disease) is primarily:
    A. increased numbers of red blood cells slowing perfusion.
    B. deficiency of surfactant increasing alveolar surface tension and causing atelectasis.
    C. right-to-left shunting of blood through a patent ductus arteriosus.
    D. epithelial cell damage causing edema.

35. A tension pneumothorax would present with:
    A. tracheal deviation and mediastinal shift away from the pneumothorax.
    B. minimal effect on blood pressure or pulse.
    C. flattened neck veins due to decreased venous return to the heart.
    D. hyperresonance to percussion and bronchial breath sounds over the uninvolved lung.

36. A pleural effusion may develop when a patient with liver disease is unable to synthesize adequate amounts of albumin. This would result in fluid movement from the vascular bed to the pleural space because of:
    A. increased pleural capillary hydrostatic pressure.
    B. increased pleural interstitial pressure.
    C. decreased pleural capillary oncotic pressure.
    D. decreased intrapleural pressure.

37. The primary feature distinguishing bacterial from viral pneumonia is:
    A. a productive cough.
    B. decreased breath sounds.
    C. atelectasis.
    D. tachycardia.

38. Transmission of Mycobacterium tuberculosis is primarily via:
    A. contaminated blood.
    B. inhaled droplets.
    C. sexual intercourse.
    D. contaminated skin that has been in contact with contaminated articles.

39. A major difference between restrictive and obstructive pulmonary diseases is that in restrictive diseases:
    A. lung tissue itself is not involved in the disease process.
    B. airway resistance is not increased.
    C. lung compliance is not altered.
    D. the inflammatory process is not a part of the pathologic condition.

40. A patient who has a large alveolar-arterial oxygen difference $(A - aDo_2)$:
    A. always has significant hypoxemia.
    B. is hypoventilating.
    C. has an enlarged zone 2 of the lung.
    D. has poor lung function and impaired gas exchange.

Fill in the Blank

41. Pulmonary hypertension is defined as a sustained increase in pulmonary artery systolic pressure above _____ mm Hg.

42. A significant increase in the resistance of the pulmonary vasculature results in pulmonary _____.

43. The three risk factors for thrombus formation commonly called Virchow's triad are _____, _____, and _____.

44. Lung cancers are rarely diagnosed before they _____ and therefore have a very low long-term survival rate.

45. The great majority of lung cancers occur in persons who _____.

46. A patient with a low V/Q usually has a reduced arterial oxygen level. The severity of the V/Q imbalance can be estimated by the difference in alveolar (PAO_2) and arterial (Pao_2) oxygen. Calculate the $A - aDo_2$ for a patient having a Pao_2 of 60 mm Hg and a $Paco_2$ of 35 mm Hg at sea level (barometric pressure = 760 mm Hg) and on room air $(FIO_2 = 0.21)$. Use an R/Q value of 0.8 and a water vapor pressure of 47 mm Hg.
    The PAO_2 is _____ mm Hg.
    The $A - aDo_2$ is _____ mm Hg.

47. The patient in the previous question is given supplemental oxygen to achieve an FIO_2 of 0.40 and his blood gases are drawn again. The Pao_2 is 100 mm Hg and the $Paco_2$ is 40 mm Hg. Calculate the $A - aDo_2$ at this time and determine if V/Q has improved:
    The PAO_2 is _____ mm Hg.
    The $A - aDo_2$ is _____ mm Hg.
    Has V/Q improved? _____

48. Regardless of the trigger for an asthma attack, all forms are characterized by airway _____, which causes mucosal edema, bronchoconstriction, and hypersecretion of mucus.

49. The increased work of breathing during an asthma attack is attributed to increased airway
_____.

50. The peak expiratory flow rate is characteristically _____ in obstructive lung disorders, but normal or _____ in restrictive disorders.

51. A patient with a significant smoking history, chronically elevated $Paco_2$, and hypoxemia most likely has a respiratory disease diagnosis of _____.

52. Diseases that cause global pulmonary hypoxemia usually are associated with pulmonary hypertension because hypoxemia causes _____ of pulmonary vessels.

53. Emphysema is a chronic obstructive disorder associated with loss of lung parenchymal tissue. Obstruction occurs because lung parenchyma is responsible for maintaining _____ _____ on the small airways.

54. A low, flat diaphragm; narrow mediastinum; and decreased lung density on chest x-ray are characteristic findings in _____.

55. Diseases that cause significant pulmonary fibrosis are associated with _____ compliance, whereas chronic obstructive pulmonary disease is associated with _____ compliance.

56. Patients with chronic obstructive pulmonary disease exert most of their work of breathing during the _____ phase of respiration, whereas those with restrictive diseases exert most of their work of breathing during the _____ phase.

57. The classic chest x-ray finding associated with pulmonary tuberculosis is a calcified nodule with a necrotic center called a _____ _____.

Case Studies

J.B. is a 46-year-old asthmatic woman who has been hospitalized with a bacterial pneumonia primarily involving the right middle and lower lobes. Antibiotics and oxygen therapy at Fio_2 0.28 by nasal cannula are initiated. A pulse oximeter is ordered to monitor oxygen saturation.

58. J.B.'s oxygen saturation is likely to be lowest when she is positioned:
    A. in a high Fowler position.
    B. lying on her left side.
    C. lying on her right side.
    D. lying supine with the head of the bed flat.

59. Using the "law of 5's," J.B.'s ideal Pao_2 level is estimated to be:
    A. 84 mm Hg.
    B. 280 mm Hg.
    C. 140 mm Hg.
    D. 28 mm Hg.

60. The combined pathophysiologic conditions of asthma and bacterial pneumonia increase the risk for J.B. to develop:
    A. hypoxemia.
    B. weakened respiratory muscles.
    C. apnea.
    D. increased residual volume.

61. Common manifestations of bacterial pneumonia include all of the following except:
    A. fever.
    B. productive cough.
    C. tachypnea.
    D. hyperinflation.

62. J.B.'s fever can be expected to alter her oxyhemoglobin desaturation curve by:
    A. shifting it to the right.
    B. shifting it to the left.
    C. inducing no change.
    D. increasing the affinity of hemoglobin for oxygen.

M.R. is a 63-year-old man who has had emphysema for many years. The nurse is on a home visit, meeting M.R. for the first time.

63. In performing a physical assessment, the nurse notes the patient has a "barrel" configuration to the chest. This is a consequence of:
    A. reduced intrapleural pressures.
    B. bronchial airway expansion.
    C. increased vital capacity.
    D. increased residual lung volume.

64. A common symptom in patients with emphysema is:
    A. nausea.
    B. significant sputum production.
    C. dyspnea.
    D. pleuritic chest pain.

65. M.R. and other patients with emphysema are at risk for which of the following complications because of the pathophysiologic process of their disease?
    A. Cancer
    B. Pneumothorax
    C. Pleural effusion
    D. Tuberculosis

66. M.R., like most patients with emphysema, is able to maintain relatively normal arterial blood gases until the disease is very advanced. This is primarily due to:
    A. secondary polycythemia.
    B. increased tidal volumes.
    C. increased respiratory effort.
    D. a slowly enlarging right side of the heart.

Five-year-old P.T. is brought to the clinic for a routine evaluation of his cystic fibrosis.

67. The underlying pathologic process of cystic fibrosis is related to:
    A. excessively thick mucus production in the lungs.
    B. decreased mucus degeneration by enzyme systems.
    C. primary surfactant deficiency.
    D. pulmonary vascular destruction.

68. Patients with cystic fibrosis are likely to develop:
    A. venous thrombi.
    B. respiratory infections.
    C. diabetes mellitus.
    D. dysrhythmias.

69. Therapeutic interventions for cystic fibrosis include all of the following except:
    A. postural drainage.
    B. nutritional supplementation.
    C. prophylactic antibiotic coverage.
    D. chloride ion supplementation.

H.J. has been hospitalized following an automobile accident. Several ribs were broken, resulting in a pneumothorax. He is being treated with a closed-chest drainage system and oxygen by nasal cannula titrated to keep his $Sao_2 \geq 90\%$.

70. Pneumothorax is:
    A. a collection of pus in the pleural space.
    B. a collection of air in the pleural space.
    C. a collection of air in alveolar blebs.
    D. a puncture in the chest wall.

71. Typical presentation of a pneumothorax includes:
    A. elevated white blood cell count.
    B. elevated blood pressure.
    C. decreased lung sounds on the affected side.
    D. increased lung sounds on the unaffected side.

72. Closed-chest drainage systems work to reexpand a lung after pneumothorax by:
    A. reestablishing the normal negative intrapleural pressure.
    B. creating a positive pressure in the pleural space.
    C. removing excess fluid from the pleural space so that there is room for lung expansion.
    D. pulling oxygen into distal air sacs to reexpand lung tissue.

Three-year-old R.C. is brought to the emergency department by her parents. They report that she seems to be having a great deal of difficulty getting a breath and has a coarse, barking cough. The nurse practitioner diagnoses croup.

73. Parents of children with croup typically report that the child has recently had:
    A. routine immunizations.
    B. an upper respiratory infection.
    C. a high fever.
    D. no recent change in health or activity.

74. Differentiation of croup from epiglottitis is essential because:
    A. they require different antibiotic therapies.
    B. croup is usually viral in origin.
    C. humidified treatments for croup will worsen epiglottitis.
    D. epiglottitis can cause rapid and complete airway obstruction.

75. Assessment findings of a child with croup include:
    A. digital clubbing.
    B. prolonged expiratory phase.
    C. expiratory wheezing.
    D. retractions of intercostal muscles with inspiration.

ANSWER KEY

ANATOMY REVIEW
Matching

1. e, a, g, h, c, i, k, d, j, b, f

NORMAL ANATOMY
AND PHYSIOLOGY REVIEW
True/False

2. T
3. F
4. F
5. T
6. T
7. F
8. F
9. F
10. T
11. T
12. T
13. F
14. T
15. T
16. T

PATHOPHYSIOLOGY QUESTIONS
Compare/Contrast

Characteristic	Chronic Bronchitis	Emphysema
Early hypoxemia	Yes	No
Early CO_2 retention	Yes	No
Productive cough	Yes	No
Increased A-P diameter	No	Yes
Cor pulmonale	Yes	No

Multiple Choice

17. A
18. C
19. D
20. A
21. B
22. B
23. C
24. A
25. D
26. A
27. A
28. B
29. C
30. C
31. D
32. A
33. C
34. B
35. A
36. C
37. A
38. B
39. B
40. D

Fill in the Blank

41. 30
42. hypertension
43. stasis of blood, hypercoagulable, injury to the vessel
44. metastasize
45. smoke cigarettes
46. $P_{AO_2} = 106$; $A - aD_{O_2} = 46$
47. $P_{AO_2} = 235$; $A - aD_{O_2} = 135$; no: the $A - aD_{O_2}$ has increased significantly
48. inflammation
49. resistance
50. decreased; increased
51. chronic bronchitis
52. vasoconstriction
53. radial traction
54. emphysema

55. low; high
56. expiratory; inspiratory
57. Ghon tubercle

Case Studies

58. C
59. C
60. A
61. D
62. A
63. D

64. C
65. B
66. C
67. A
68. B
69. D
70. B
71. C
72. A
73. B
74. D
75. D

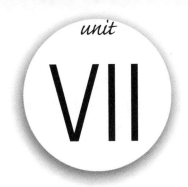

Fluid, Electrolyte, and Acid-Base Homeostasis

Chapters 24 and 25

NORMAL ANATOMY AND PHYSIOLOGY REVIEW
True/False

Indicate whether each of the following statements regarding the anatomy and physiology of fluid-electrolyte and acid-base balance is true (T) or false (F).

1. _____ The principal regulators of fluid intake are thirst and habit.

2. _____ Fluid movement across the capillary wall is determined by filtration pressure.

3. _____ Electrolyte movement across the capillary wall is determined by diffusion.

4. _____ The principal determinant of capillary filtration is interstitial hydrostatic pressure.

5. _____ Osmosis is an active, energy-requiring process.

6. _____ Water moves across cell membranes according to osmotic gradients.

7. _____ Two-thirds of the total body fluid is contained in the extracellular space.

8. _____ When isotonic fluids are administered, they remain in the extracellular space and do not enter the cells.

9. _____ When water is administered, it distributes among all fluid compartments by osmosis.

10. _____ Aldosterone is a hormone that promotes reabsorption of water in the collecting tubule.

11. _____ Antidiuretic hormone (ADH) induces the kidney to produce concentrated urine.

12. _____ The normal ratio of bicarbonate to carbonic acid is 10:1.

13. _____ A pH buffer releases H^+ when pH is high and binds H^+ when pH is low.

14. _____ The bicarbonate buffer system is the most important pH buffer in the extracellular fluid.

15. _____ The kidneys control the level of bicarbonate in the extracellular fluid.

Laboratory Values

Evaluate the following laboratory values and write N for normal, H for abnormally high, and L for abnormally low.

16. _____ Serum potassium: 3.8 mEq/L

17. _____ $Paco_2$: 30 mm Hg

18. _____ Arterial pH: 7.38

19. _____ Serum calcium: 9.5 mg/dl

20. _____ Serum sodium: 149 mEq/L

21. _____ Arterial HCO_3^-: 24 mEq/L

22. _____ Serum Mg^{2+}: 6.0 mEq/L

PATHOPHYSIOLOGY QUESTIONS
Compare/Contrast

Compare and contrast electrolyte disorders by filling in the following tables.

Characteristic	Hypernatremia	Hyponatremia
Etiologic factor		
Clinical findings		
Treatment		

Characteristic	Hyperkalemia	Hypokalemia
Etiologic factor		
Clinical findings		
Treatment		

Characteristic	Hypercalcemia	Hypocalcemia
Etiologic factor		
Clinical findings		
Treatment		

Characteristic	Hypermagnesemia	Hypomagnesemia
Etiologic factor		
Clinical findings		
Treatment		

Characteristic	Hyperphosphatemia	Hypophosphatemia
Etiologic factor		
Clinical findings		
Treatment		

Multiple Choice

Select the one best answer to each of the following questions.

23. Saline deficit is defined as:
    A. a deficit of extracellular volume.
    B. a deficit of serum sodium.
    C. a deficit of body water.
    D. hyponatremia.

24. Signs and symptoms of saline deficit include:
    A. low serum sodium.
    B. increased serum osmolality.
    C. postural hypotension.
    D. seizures.

25. Water excess (hyponatremia) is best detected by:
    A. weight changes.
    B. blood pressure changes.
    C. low serum sodium.
    D. edema.

26. Conditions that predispose to hyponatremia include:
    A. high rates of isotonic fluid administration.
    B. significant blood loss.
    C. insufficient production of ADH.
    D. excessive administration of 5% dextrose in water (D_5W).

27. If a patient with a normal serum sodium is given 1 L of normal saline, how much of that volume will distribute into the intracellular space?
    A. None
    B. One third
    C. Two thirds
    D. All

28. If a patient is given 1 L of D_5W, how much of that volume will distribute to the intracellular space?
    A. None
    B. One third
    C. Two thirds
    D. All

29. The most appropriate fluid for treating a patient with a normal serum sodium and an extracellular volume deficit is:
    A. whole blood.
    B. isotonic fluid (e.g., normal saline).
    C. D_5W.
    D. unrestricted oral water.

30. Generalized edema is usually a consequence of:
    A. excessive extracellular volume.
    B. reduced plasma proteins.
    C. high blood pressure.
    D. increased capillary hydrostatic pressure.

31. Dependent edema is usually a consequence of:
    A. hyponatremia.
    B. reduced plasma proteins.
    C. high arterial blood pressure.
    D. increased capillary hydrostatic pressure.

32. The plasma concentration of an electrolyte correlates most closely with:
    A. the intracellular concentration.
    B. the interstitial concentration.
    C. the urinary concentration.
    D. the cerebrospinal fluid concentration.

33. Muscle weakness may be a symptom of all of the following electrolyte disturbances except:
    A. hyperkalemia.
    B. hypercalcemia.
    C. hypermagnesemia.
    D. hyperphosphatemia.

34. Manifestations of potassium imbalance are attributed to:
    A. altered threshold for excitation.
    B. altered resting membrane potential.
    C. altered release of neurotransmitter at the neuromuscular junction.
    D. altered production of intracellular ATP.

35. Manifestations of magnesium imbalance are attributed to:
    A. altered threshold for excitation.
    B. altered resting membrane potential.
    C. altered release of neurotransmitter at the neuromuscular junction.
    D. altered production of intracellular ATP.

36. Manifestations of calcium imbalance are attributed to:
    A. altered threshold for excitation.
    B. altered resting membrane potential.
    C. altered release of neurotransmitter at the neuromuscular junction.
    D. altered production of intracellular ATP.

37. The role of the lungs in maintaining acid-base balance includes:
    A. elimination of metabolic acids.
    B. elimination of excess H^+.
    C. production of bicarbonate.
    D. elimination of carbonic acid.

38. In response to a chronically elevated $Paco_2$, the kidneys would be expected to compensate by:
    A. excreting more bicarbonate.
    B. producing more bicarbonate.
    C. reabsorbing more hydrogen ions.
    D. filtering more bicarbonate.

39. Which of the following arterial blood gases would be categorized as compensated metabolic acidosis?
    A. pH 7.39, $Paco_2$ 32, HCO_3^- 18
    B. pH 7.31, $Paco_2$ 37, HCO_3^- 18
    C. pH 7.45, $Paco_2$ 32, HCO_3^- 23
    D. pH 7.40, $Paco_2$ 39, HCO_3^- 24

40. A blood gas with pH 7.24, $Paco_2$ 58, HCO_3^- 24 would be categorized as:
    A. metabolic acidosis.
    B. metabolic alkalosis.
    C. respiratory acidosis.
    D. respiratory alkalosis.

Fill in the Blank

41. A patient exhibiting edema, weight gain, and a normal serum sodium level probably has a fluid imbalance called _____.

42. Hypernatremia and increased serum osmolality are associated with a deficit of _____.

43. A normal serum potassium is between _____ and _____ mEq/L.

44. A high serum potassium causes the resting membrane potential to be _____, whereas a low serum potassium _____ the resting membrane potential.

45. While having his blood pressure taken with a cuff inflated around the upper arm, the patient complains of tingling and spasms of the hand. These symptoms are called a positive _____ sign and usually are a consequence of _____ or _____.

46. A patient who presents with unexplained hypercalcemia should be evaluated for _____ as the cause.

47. When a pregnant woman with preeclampsia is given a magnesium infusion to suppress seizures during delivery, one should anticipate that the newborn may exhibit _____.

48. A normal blood pH can be maintained despite variances in HCO_3^- and carbonic acid as long as their ratio is maintained at _____.

49. The amount of H^+ excreted in the urine can be increased by combining the H^+ with urine buffers in the following reactions: _____; _____.

50. In general, acidosis produces central nervous system _____ and alkalosis produces central nervous system _____.

Case Studies

Joe is a 24-year-old man brought to the emergency department by a friend. The friend reports that Joe spent the day on the lake in a boat and then developed severe headache and vomiting in the evening. He has been unable to keep down any fluids, and he is warm and flushed with a temperature of 102° F. He has not urinated in the last 16 hours.

51. Joe's blood pressure is 90/50 and his heart rate is 118 beats/minute when he is supine. When at the nurse's request he attempts to sit up for an orthostatic blood pressure reading, he becomes faint and must lie down. These findings are consistent with a diagnosis of:
    A. saline deficit.
    B. hyponatremia.
    C. renal failure.
    D. cardiogenic shock.

52. Laboratory analysis of Joe's blood reveals that his serum sodium is 150 mEq/L, indicating:
    A. saline excess.
    B. water deficit.
    C. hyponatremia.
    D. a normal value.

53. An intravenous line is established to provide fluid replacement. The most appropriate fluid for expanding Joe's extracellular volume to improve his blood pressure and heart rate is:
    A. water.
    B. 5% dextrose in water.
    C. normal saline (0.9%).
    D. half-normal saline (0.045%).

54. Joe received 3 L of isotonic fluid, and his blood pressure stabilized at 110/70 with a heart rate of 80 beats/min while he was supine. When Joe stood up, his blood pressure dropped to 100/60 with a heart rate of 96 beats/min. This indicates that:
    A. Joe has received adequate fluid replacement therapy.
    B. Joe's intravenous fluid should be changed to a hypotonic fluid.
    C. Joe needs more isotonic fluid replacement.
    D. Joe is not responding to fluid therapy.

55. For which acid-base disorder is Joe at risk if his vomiting continues for a prolonged period?
    A. Respiratory acidosis
    B. Respiratory alkalosis
    C. Metabolic acidosis
    D. Metabolic alkalosis

Cindy is a 16-year-old girl with type 1 (insulin-dependent) diabetes. In addition to her morning and evening doses of insulin, she is to monitor her blood glucose four times daily and supplement the insulin as needed. For the past several weeks Cindy has been extremely busy with school activities and has not been monitoring her blood glucose carefully. She is now in the clinic complaining of severe fatigue and abdominal pain.

56. A urine sample reveals the presence of ketones. What acid-base disorder may accompany excessive ketone production?
    A. Respiratory acidosis
    B. Respiratory alkalosis
    C. Metabolic acidosis
    D. Metabolic alkalosis

57. An arterial blood gas is obtained, which shows pH 7.38, Pa_{CO_2} 33, and HCO_3^- 19. This blood gas is consistent with a diagnosis of:
    A. compensated metabolic acidosis.
    B. uncompensated metabolic acidosis.
    C. compensated respiratory alkalosis.
    D. uncompensated respiratory alkalosis.

58. What action would be most appropriate at this time to manage this acid-base disorder?
    A. Manage the underlying problem with insulin.
    B. Administer sodium bicarbonate to normalize the HCO_3^-.
    C. Have the patient breathe into a paper bag to normalize the Pa_{CO_2}.
    D. Do nothing; this is a normal blood gas.

59. An electrolyte disorder that often accompanies diabetic ketosis is:
   A. hyponatremia.
   B. hypochloremia.
   C. hyperkalemia.
   D. hypophosphatemia.

60. A finger stick blood glucose sample shows a value of 336 mg/dl, and there is significant glycosuria. These two findings suggest that Cindy likely has a deficit of:
   A. sodium bicarbonate.
   B. potassium.
   C. urine output.
   D. fluid volume.

NORMAL ANATOMY AND PHYSIOLOGY REVIEW
True/False

1. T
2. T
3. T
4. F
5. F
6. T
7. F
8. T
9. T
10. F
11. T
12. F
13. T
14. T
15. T

Laboratory Values

16. N
17. L
18. N
19. N
20. H
21. N
22. H

PATHOPHYSIOLOGY QUESTIONS
Compare/Contrast

Characteristic	Hypernatremia	Hyponatremia

Etiologic factor	Chronic diarrhea
	Restricted access to fluid
	Altered thirst sensation
	Diabetes insipidus
	Diabetes mellitus
	Fevers
		Excess hypotonic IV fluid
		Excess ADH (SIADH)
		Excess water intake:
		  Tap water enemas
		  NG irrigation with water
		Psychogenic polydipsia

Clinical findings	High serum sodium High serum osmolality Confusion, lethargy, convulsions owing to cellular shriveling	Low serum sodium Low serum osmolality Confusion, lethargy, nausea, coma, convulsions owing to cellular swelling
Treatment	Increase free water intake Hypotonic IV fluids Treat slowly to avoid rebound cellular swelling	Free water restriction Avoid hypotonic IV fluid Perhaps diuretics Can give hypertonic IV solutions cautiously

Characteristic	Hyperkalemia	Hypokalemia

Etiologic factor	Increased intake:
	    Accidental IV bolus
	    Salt substitute
	    Administration of older units of blood
	Decreased excretion:
	    Oliguric renal failure
	    Low aldosterone
	Shift from body cells:
	    Crushing injuries
	    Acidosis
	    Chemotherapy
		Decreased intake:
		    NPO status
		Anorexia, vomiting
		Increased excretion:
		    Diuretics
		    High aldosterone
		    Diarrhea, vomiting
		    Nasogastric suction
		Shift into body cells:
		    Alkalosis
		    Glucose/insulin infusion

Clinical findings	Muscle weakness Ascending paralysis Cardiac dysrhythmias	Muscle weakness, cramps Paralytic ileus Cardiac dysrhythmias
Treatment	Dialysis Sodium polystyrene sulfonate (Kayexalate) Insulin/glucose Correct acidosis if present	IV or PO potassium replacement Correct alkalosis if present

Characteristic	Hypercalcemia	Hypocalcemia

Etiologic factor	Increased intake:
	    Excessive antacids
	    Excessive vitamin D
	Decreased excretion:
	    Hyperparathyroidism
	Shift from body cells:
	    Immobility
	    Hyperparathyroidism
	    Malignancy
		Decreased intake:
		    Malabsorption syndrome
		    Milk intolerance
		Increased excretion:
		    Chronic renal insufficiency
		    Hypoparathyroidism
		Shift out of blood:
		    Massive blood transfusion (citrate
		    binding)

Clinical findings	Muscle weakness
	Constipation
	CNS depression
		Muscle cramping, twitching, tetany:
		    + Chvostek sign
		    + Trousseau sign
		Convulsions, laryngospasm

Treatment	Increased fluid intake Manage underlying cause: Parathyroidectomy tumor resection Diuretics	IV or PO calcium supplementation

Characteristic	Hypermagnesemia	Hypomagnesemia
Etiologic factor	Excessive antacid intake IV infusion for pregnancy-induced hypertension Renal failure	Malabsorption syndrome Alcoholism Diuretics
Clinical findings	Muscle weakness Decreased deep tendon reflexes Similar to hypercalcemia	Muscle cramping, twitching: + Chvostek sign + Trousseau sign Similar to hypocalcemia
Treatment	Increased fluid intake Diuretics	IV or PO magnesium replacement

Characteristic	Hyperphosphatemia	Hypophosphatemia
Etiology	Renal failure	Chronic alcoholism Refeeding after starvation High glucose solutions (TPN)
Clinical findings	Precipitation of $CaPO_4$ salts in organs, joints, vessels, etc. Often associated with hypocalcemia	May have multisystem signs and symptoms because of cellular energy failure: phosphate is needed for ATP synthesis
Treatment	Phosphate-binding antacids Diuretics Measures to increase calcium absorption	IV or PO phosphate replacement

Multiple Choice

23. A
24. C
25. C
26. D
27. A
28. C
29. B
30. B
31. D
32. B
33. D
34. B
35. C
36. A
37. D
38. B
39. A
40. C

Fill in the Blank

41. saline excess (extracellular volume excess)
42. water
43. 3.5, 5.0
44. hypopolarized, hyperpolarized
45. Trousseau; hypocalcemia; hypomagnesemia
46. cancer (malignancy)
47. neuromuscular and respiratory muscle weakness
48. 20:1
49. $NH_3 + H^+ \rightarrow NH_4^+$; $HPO_4^{2-} + H^+ \rightarrow H_2PO_4^-$
50. depression, excitation

Case Studies

51. A
52. B
53. C
54. C
55. D

56. C
57. A
58. A
59. C
60. D

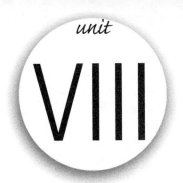

unit
VIII

Renal and Bladder Function

Chapters 26 to 29

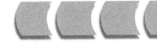

ANATOMY REVIEW
Matching

1. Match each lettered item in the figure with one of the following anatomic terms:

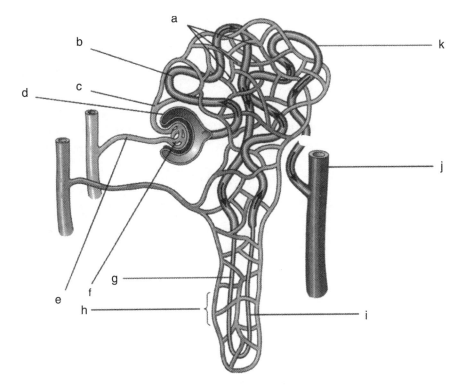

_____ Afferent arteriole

_____ Efferent arteriole

_____ Ascending loop of Henle

_____ Collecting tubule

_____ Proximal convoluted tubule

_____ Descending loop of Henle

_____ Glomerulus

_____ Bowman capsule

_____ Peritubular capillaries

_____ Vasa recta

_____ Distal convoluted tubule

NORMAL ANATOMY AND PHYSIOLOGY REVIEW
Matching

Match the terms in the right column with their definitions in the left column.

2. _____ The functional unit of the kidney

3. _____ Percentage of the cardiac output delivered to the kidneys

4. _____ External landmark for the location of the kidneys

5. _____ Area of the kidney where the glomeruli and nephron tubules are located

6. _____ Area of the kidney receiving the smallest amount of blood

7. _____ Branch of the autonomic nervous system that controls intrarenal perfusion and the release of renin

8. _____ The movement of fluid from an area of higher pressure to an area of lower pressure; occurs in the glomerulus

9. _____ Area of the kidney where two thirds of the water and electrolytes are reabsorbed into the blood

10. _____ Area of the kidney where aldosterone acts to produce sodium and water reabsorption

11. _____ Area of the kidney where water is reabsorbed under the influence of antidiuretic hormone

12. _____ Loss of large molecules such as protein and blood cells is prevented by this

13. _____ Renal participation in acid-base balance is primarily through secretion of _____ and reabsorption and generation of _____

14. _____ Potassium balance is primarily controlled by the action of this hormone

15. _____ This hormone inhibits the effects of aldosterone, resulting in sodium and water elimination from the body

16. _____ Hypoxia causes the release of this hormone from the kidney

17. _____ Renal activation of this will allow absorption of dietary calcium

18. _____ Laboratory test that best reflects glomerular filtration rate (GFR)

19. _____ Laboratory test affected by the hydration status and metabolic rate of the patient

A. atrial natriuretic peptide
B. 50%
C. basement membrane
D. secretion
E. medulla
F. vitamin D
G. aldosterone
H. nephron
I. 20%
J. serum creatinine
K. parasympathetic nervous system
L. proximal convoluted tubule
M. HPO_4^{2-}; NH_3
N. erythropoietin
O. costovertebral angle
P. distal convoluted tubule
Q. H^+; HCO_3^-
R. BUN
S. sympathetic nervous system
T. retroperitoneal
U. filtration
V. excretion
W. collecting ducts
X. cortex
Y. renal pelvis
Z. renal biopsy

PATHOPHYSIOLOGY QUESTIONS
Compare/Contrast

Compare and contrast cystitis and pyelonephritis by filling in the following table. Write "yes" or "no" in the appropriate columns.

Characteristic	Cystitis	Pyelonephritis
Frequency, urgency, and dysuria		
Increased serum WBC		
Flank pain		
Fever		
Costovertebral angle tenderness		
Urinary casts		

True/False

Indicate whether the following statements are true (T) or false (F).

20. _____ The most common inherited congenital renal disorder is renal agenesis.

21. _____ A tumor in the bladder could produce postrenal failure.

22. _____ One risk factor for the development of renal failure is simply aging.

23. _____ Stress incontinence is due to inappropriate stimulation of the parasympathetic nervous system.

24. _____ Secretions from the prostate gland help to protect men from urinary tract infections.

25. _____ Stones forming in the urinary bladder are usually composed of calcium.

26. _____ A person who develops nephrolithiasis has a better than 50% chance of experiencing another episode.

27. _____ The majority of tumors affecting the kidney are malignant.

28. _____ Cystitis typically presents with dysuria, frequency, and urgency.

29. _____ A common finding in the urinalysis of a patient with acute tubular necrosis (ATN) is increased protein and red blood cells.

30. _____ Nephrotic syndrome is a result of any condition that causes large amounts of protein to pass into the filtrate at the glomerular basement membrane.

31. _____ Pregnant women with cystitis are aggressively treated because of the increased risk of developing pyelonephritis.

32. _____ Elevated BUN values seen in chronic and acute renal failure are due to volume reduction during the diuretic phase.

33. _____ Spinal cord injury results in a loss of voluntary bladder control, called a neurogenic bladder.

34. _____ Acute renal failure normally progresses through three phases in the following order: oliguric, diuretic, and recovery phase.

Multiple Choice

Select the one best answer to each of the following questions.

35. Polycystic renal disease:
    A. is associated with impaired function of the gallbladder and pancreas in children.
    B. manifests with decreasing renal function, hypertension, and flank pain in adults.
    C. is seen as small, atrophied kidneys on sonogram.
    D. is very responsive to treatment and ultimately curable.

36. The most common cause of urinary tract infections is:
    A. gram-negative organisms such as *E. coli, Pseudomonas,* and *Proteus.*
    B. gram-positive organisms such as *Staphylococcus.*
    C. fungal organisms.
    D. viral organisms.

37. Pyelonephritis can be differentiated from cystitis by:
    A. presence of dysuria, frequency, and urgency.
    B. the causative organism.
    C. bladder tenderness with palpation.
    D. fever, flank pain, and WBC casts in the urine.

38. The most common component of renal calculi (pyelocalculi) is:
    A. calcium.
    B. uric acid.
    C. cystine.
    D. struvite.

39. Nephroblastoma or Wilms tumor is the most common renal malignancy in children. Its diagnosis is:
    A. followed by aggressive chemotherapy as the primary intervention.
    B. made on the basis of an abnormal urinalysis result.
    C. often suggested by a palpable mass in the flank or abdomen.
    D. grave because the prognosis is very poor in all cases.

40. Acute glomerulonephritis:
    A. relentlessly progresses to chronic renal failure.
    B. presents with the classic signs and symptoms of fluid volume deficit and increased plasma oncotic pressure.
    C. is usually a result of an antigen-antibody reaction.
    D. produces a pathologic increase in GFR.

41. In addition to glomerulonephritis, another common cause of nephrotic syndrome is:
    A. diabetes.
    B. recurrent urinary tract infections.
    C. urinary obstruction.
    D. renal tumors.

42. The etiologic difference between acute and chronic glomerulonephritis is:
    A. the specific organism causing the infection.
    B. the chronic form is usually autoimmune, whereas the acute form results from an immune reaction to infection.
    C. the chronic form is attributable to a slowly declining GFR.
    D. not of any assistance because the cause is the same, but the acute form progresses more quickly.

43. Pain in the kidney, as occurs with pyelonephritis or trauma, is a result of:
    A. the presence of abundant nociceptors throughout the kidney tissue.
    B. irritation of densely packed pain receptors in the renal pelvis.
    C. activation of afferent nerves of the corticospinal tracts.
    D. stimulation of pain receptors located in the renal capsule.

44. Obstruction of a ureter by a calculus may produce significant changes in the kidney, including:
    A. a rapid and significant reduction in renal perfusion.
    B. atrophy of the renal pelvis.
    C. maintenance of GFR through autoregulation.
    D. patches of ischemic tissue.

45. Prerenal failure, regardless of the specific cause, has a single common etiologic factor, which is:
    A. inactivation of the renal autoregulatory mechanisms.
    B. narrowing of afferent arterioles.
    C. a reduction in renal perfusion.
    D. decreased effect of aldosterone and antidiuretic hormones.

46. All of the following could produce prerenal failure except:
    A. myocardial infarction.
    B. pyelonephritis.
    C. septic shock.
    D. hemorrhage.

47. Damage to the kidney from nephrotoxic drugs:
    A. is irreversible.
    B. affects the epithelial cells of the renal tubules.
    C. impairs glomerular basement membrane permeability.
    D. commonly progresses to end-stage renal disease.

48. Back leak of filtrate, an important aspect of the pathologic development of ATN:
    A. contributes to retention of creatinine in the blood.
    B. forces efferent and afferent arterioles to vasodilate.
    C. is due to dilation of renal tubules.
    D. increases platelet aggregation and the risk of thrombosis formation.

49. Acute renal failure produces all of the following characteristic alterations in laboratory values except:
    A. elevated serum creatinine.
    B. azotemia.
    C. uremia.
    D. decreased serum potassium.

50. The stage of chronic renal failure known as "decreased renal reserve":
    A. produces polyuria and nocturia.
    B. presents as mild azotemia.
    C. is asymptomatic.
    D. can be diagnosed only by elevated serum creatinine and BUN.

51. Findings associated with chronic renal failure but not likely to be found with acute renal failure include:
    A. elevations in serum creatinine and BUN.
    B. fluid volume excess.
    C. hypocalcemia and anemia.
    D. metabolic acidosis.

52. Renal insufficiency:
    A. may be controlled with dietary management.
    B. requires intervention with dialysis or renal transplantation.
    C. is associated with a nephron loss of about 50%.
    D. is successfully managed with diuretic therapy.

53. Which of the following patients is at highest risk for developing prerenal acute renal failure?
    A. An elderly patient with benign prostatic hyperplasia.
    B. A young woman with acute pyelonephritis.
    C. An elderly woman receiving nephrotoxic antibiotics.
    D. A young man with significant postsurgical hemorrhage.

54. Regardless of the type, all forms of dialysis have in common:
    A. significant risk for volume overload.
    B. a synthetic, artificial membrane between the bloodstream and dialysate fluid.
    C. removal of blood from the body for processing by dialysis.
    D. removal of excess electrolytes and wastes by diffusion.

55. For most patients receiving dialysis therapy, the dialysate composition is designed to:
    A. remove serum calcium.
    B. remove serum potassium.
    C. increase serum phosphate.
    D. increase extracellular fluid volume.

56. Nocturnal enuresis in children is:
    A. always pathologic after the age of 5 years.
    B. nearly always managed with pharmacologic interventions.
    C. most commonly due to maturational delay.
    D. frequently associated with daytime enuresis.

57. The most common cause of bladder calculi is:
    A. urinary tract infection.
    B. urinary retention and stasis.
    C. increased dietary calcium intake.
    D. reduced GFR.

58. Risk factors for the development of cystitis include all of the following except:
    A. female gender.
    B. acidic urine.
    C. urinary stasis.
    D. diabetes mellitus.

59. Cystitis is:
    A. an inflammation of the bladder lining.
    B. always associated with bacterial infection.
    C. a common cause of renal failure.
    D. always symptomatic.

60. Bladder tumors:
    A. are most commonly formed in the musculature of the bladder wall.
    B. are always associated with exposure to carcinogens.
    C. are more common among African-Americans.
    D. may present with occult or macroscopic hematuria.

61. Vesicoureteral reflux, a congenital malformation, is usually diagnosed by:
    A. decreased frequency of voiding.
    B. an enlarged kidney found on abdominal x-ray film.
    C. complaints of flank pain.
    D. incidence of recurrent urinary tract infection.

62. The most common obstruction of the urinary tract found in children is ureteropelvic junction obstruction. This condition is:
    A. hereditary in origin.
    B. usually bilateral, affecting both ureters.
    C. usually diagnosed by ultrasound in utero.
    D. likely to resolve spontaneously.

63. Congenital malformations of the ureters primarily produce signs and symptoms related to:
    A. abnormal bladder distention.
    B. elevations in BUN and serum creatinine.
    C. urinary stasis.
    D. renal atrophy.

Fill in the Blank

64. A normal urinalysis may contain up to _____ RBCs or WBCs per high-powered field.

65. The presence of urinary casts is helpful in diagnosing certain kidney diseases: _____ casts signify pyelonephritis; _____ casts signify glomerulonephritis; and _____ casts signify tubular necrosis and sloughing of tubule cells.

66. Most renal calculi are composed of _____.

67. A child presenting with periorbital edema and hematuria should be evaluated for _____.

68. Diabetic nephropathy should be suspected in diabetic patients who have _____ in their urine.

69. Plasmapheresis may be used to manage certain types of glomerulonephritis in which renal damage is caused by _____.

70. Postrenal acute renal failure is caused by processes that _____.

71. The phases of chronic renal failure include an asymptomatic phase that lasts until about _____% of nephron function is lost.

72. End-stage renal disease and uremia occur when GFR falls below about _____% of normal.

73. Patients with chronic renal failure usually have a normocytic, normochromic anemia owing to lack of _____.

74. The diagnostic test used to determine the GFR in an individual is _____.

75. Patients with chronic renal failure may be asked to restrict their protein intake because protein is a source of _____ wastes and may worsen azotemia.

Case Studies

T.G. comes to the nurse practitioner clinic complaining of burning during urination, as well as a feeling of needing to urinate more often than usual. She is a 25-year-old graduate student and has recently returned from her honeymoon.

76. The symptoms T.G. reports are characteristic of:
    A. a bladder tumor.
    B. enuresis.
    C. bladder calculi.
    D. cystitis.

77. In order to confirm the diagnosis, the nurse practitioner orders:
    A. a urinalysis.
    B. an intravenous pyelogram.
    C. an abdominal x-ray film.
    D. an abdominal ultrasound.

78. Results of this diagnostic test that support the preliminary diagnosis would be:
    A. radiopaque stones visible in the bladder.
    B. obstructed renal perfusion.
    C. bacteria in the urine.
    D. an abdominal mass.

79. The appropriate intervention for the nurse practitioner to initiate would be:
    A. a standard course of antibiotic therapy.
    B. renal ultrasound to evaluate for pyelonephritis.
    C. referral to a surgeon.
    D. referral to a nephrologist.

80. Counseling that the nurse practitioner would provide for T.G. would also likely include all of the following except:
   A. increased fluid intake.
   B. abstinence from sexual intercourse.
   C. urination following sexual intercourse.
   D. correct cleansing technique following bowel movements.

Sixty-five-year-old C.V. was admitted to the hospital for management of dehydration associated with a severe gastrointestinal flu.

81. What type of acute renal failure is C.V. at risk for?
   A. Prerenal
   B. Postrenal
   C. Pyelonephritis
   D. Glomerulonephritis

82. Indeed, C.V. does develop prerenal oliguria. Which of the following would not be found among her laboratory results?
   A. Low urinary sodium levels
   B. BUN/creatinine ratio greater than 20:1
   C. Low urine specific gravity
   D. High urine osmolality

83. The appropriate intervention for the prerenal oliguria phase of C.V.'s disorder would be:
   A. dialysis.
   B. extracellular volume expansion.
   C. monitoring serum BUN and limiting protein intake.
   D. aggressive diuretic therapy.

84. Improvement in C.V.'s GFR correlates most closely with:
   A. normalizing of serum creatinine levels.
   B. normalizing of BUN.
   C. normalizing of urine specific gravity.
   D. normalizing of albumin levels.

85. C.V. responds poorly to therapy and enters the oliguric phase of acute renal failure. When this occurs:
   A. tubular casts may be found in the urine.
   B. hematuria may ensue.
   C. an increase in urinary output is expected.
   D. the concentration of sodium in the urine declines.

A.P. is a 56-year-old man who is being treated for chronic pyelonephritis. He is currently living in a homeless shelter, but when the weather warms in the spring, he typically "moves outside somewhere."

86. The cause of chronic pyelonephritis is:
   A. prostatic hypertrophy.
   B. glomerulonephritis.
   C. recurrent urinary infections.
   D. failure to respond to the urge to void.

87. The health care workers are concerned about A.P. because chronic pyelonephritis is:
    A. a premalignant condition.
    B. a common cause of cystitis.
    C. a cause of significant fluid and electrolyte abnormalities.
    D. a leading cause of renal failure.

88. Careful, thorough teaching will be necessary because:
    A. A.P. is not likely to have access to hygienic bathroom facilities.
    B. a balanced diet and increased protein intake are essential.
    C. A.P. is not likely to void on a regular basis.
    D. antibiotic therapy must be continued for a prolonged course.

Arriving in the emergency department in acute pain, 20-year-old M.N. is on the edge of tears. He says the pain began when he was sitting in his college class, nearly causing him to double over. He tells the triage nurse that it "just came on—bang, and it just gets worse." He rates his pain as 10 out of 10, stating that it is located low and to the left of his spine. It seems to "come in waves."

89. M.N.'s description is classic for renal colic associated with renal calculi. Other associated signs or symptoms typically include:
    A. nausea and vomiting.
    B. decreased urinary output.
    C. enuresis.
    D. diarrhea.

90. Most renal calculi are initially evaluated with a/an:
    A. urine culture.
    B. X-ray film of the kidneys, ureters, and bladder.
    C. serum creatinine and BUN.
    D. CT scan.

91. It is determined that M.N.'s calculi are small (<5 mm) and so should pass in his urine. Treatment at this time will include:
    A. bed rest.
    B. hospitalization and intravenous fluids.
    C. NPO and antiemetics.
    D. analgesics and increased fluids.

Seven-year-old L.E. has developed acute glomerulonephritis following a strep throat infection. Fortunately, he was a healthy boy before this, so his physician and family are optimistic that he will make a full recovery.

92. If acute glomerulonephritis progresses to renal failure, what type of renal failure will it cause?
    A. Prerenal
    B. Intrarenal
    C. ATN
    D. Postrenal

93. L.E. begins to have significant proteinuria, and a 24-hour urine collection contains 4.0 g of protein. L.E. has progressed to:
    A. renal failure.
    B. ATN.
    C. needing dialysis.
    D. nephrosis.

94. The loss of significant protein in the urine contributes to all of the following manifestations except:
    A. edema.
    B. ascites.
    C. hematuria.
    D. effusions in the pleural space.

95. The key therapy for preventing poststreptococcal acute glomerulonephritis is:
    A. antibiotic therapy for streptococcal pharyngitis.
    B. avoidance of antipyretics during acute pharyngitis.
    C. prophylactic antibiotics during the school year.
    D. administration of antistreptococcal antibodies to susceptible individuals.

The nurses working in the outpatient hemodialysis unit are very familiar with B.J. He has been receiving dialysis treatments for chronic renal failure three times a week for 4 years. He is 44 years old and works as an accountant. The cause of his chronic renal failure is diabetes, which he has had since the age of 11 years.

96. When B.J. comes in for treatment, he usually has some of the signs and symptoms of fluid volume overload (especially if he ate potato chips the night before!). All of the following would be seen except:
    A. rales in the bases of the lungs.
    B. 2+ edema of the ankles.
    C. jugular venous distention.
    D. faint peripheral pulses.

97. Patients with chronic renal failure usually exhibit:
    A. bradycardia.
    B. hypokalemia.
    C. hypocalcemia.
    D. hematomas.

98. B.J. is at risk for some problems because of his chronic renal failure that do not occur with acute renal failure. These include:
    A. osteodystrophy.
    B. metabolic acidosis.
    C. elevated serum potassium.
    D. azotemia.

99. Chronic renal failure is:
    A. a reversible disorder.
    B. a progressive disorder.
    C. a disorder with an unpredictable course.
    D. a disorder that spontaneously improves with time.

100. The diet of a patient in renal failure is restricted in all of the following except:
     A. fluid.
     B. potassium.
     C. protein.
     D. calories.

ANATOMY
Matching

1. e, c, i, j, b, g, f, d, a, h, k

NORMAL ANATOMY
AND PHYSIOLOGY REVIEW
Matching

2. H
3. I
4. O
5. X
6. E

7. S
8. U
9. L
10. P
11. W
12. C
13. Q
14. G
15. A
16. N
17. F
18. J
19. R

PATHOPHYSIOLOGY QUESTIONS
Compare/Contrast

Characteristic	Cystitis	Pyelonephritis
Frequency, urgency, and dysuria	Yes	Yes
Increased serum WBC	No	Yes
Flank pain	No	Yes
Fever	No	Yes
Costovertebral angle tenderness	No	Yes
Urinary casts	No	Yes

True/False

20. F
21. T
22. T
23. F
24. T
25. F
26. T
27. T
28. T
29. F
30. T
31. T
32. F
33. T
34. T

Multiple Choice

35. B
36. A
37. D
38. A
39. C
40. C
41. A
42. B
43. D
44. D
45. C
46. B
47. B
48. A
49. D

50. C
51. C
52. A
53. D
54. D
55. B
56. C
57. B
58. B
59. A
60. D
61. D
62. C
63. C

Fill in the Blank

64. 5
65. WBC; RBC; tubular epithelial
66. calcium
67. glomerulonephritis
68. protein
69. antibodies
70. obstruct urine flow distal to the kidneys
71. 75
72. 10
73. erythropoietin
74. creatinine (or inulin) clearance rate
75. nitrogenous

Case Studies

76. D
77. A
78. C
79. A
80. B
81. A
82. C
83. B
84. A
85. A
86. C
87. D
88. D
89. A
90. B
91. D
92. B
93. D
94. C
95. A
96. D
97. C
98. A
99. B
100. D

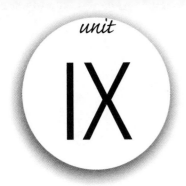
Genital and Reproductive Function

Chapters 30 to 34

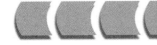

ANATOMY REVIEW
Matching

1. Match each lettered item in the figure with one of the following anatomic terms:

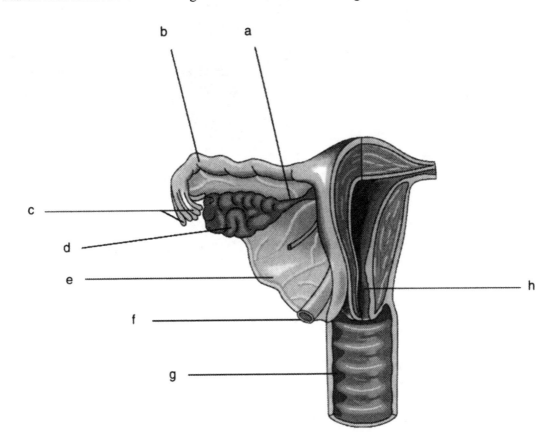

_____ Fallopian tube   _____ Fimbria

_____ Broad ligament   _____ Ovarian ligament

_____ Uterus   _____ Vagina

_____ Ovary   _____ Uterosacral ligament

2. Match each lettered item in the figure with one of the following anatomic terms:

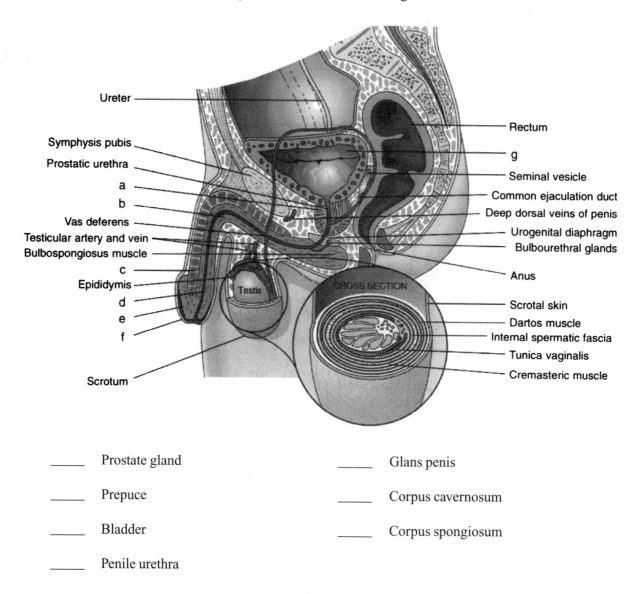

_____ Prostate gland   _____ Glans penis

_____ Prepuce   _____ Corpus cavernosum

_____ Bladder   _____ Corpus spongiosum

_____ Penile urethra

NORMAL ANATOMY AND PHYSIOLOGY REVIEW
True/False

Indicate whether the following statements regarding the anatomy and physiology of the genital and reproductive system are true (T) or false (F).

3. _____ Movement of urine through the ureters is facilitated by smooth muscle contractions.

4. _____ The epididymis is the area of the testes where sperm are produced.

5. _____ Penile erection is mediated by the sympathetic nervous system.

6. _____ External genitalia development begins at the sixth week of fetal development.

7. _____ Normal bladder capacity is 450 to 500 ml.

8. _____ Endometrial proliferation is enhanced by the hormone progesterone.

9. _____ Release of milk from the breast tissue ducts is mediated by oxytocin from the posterior pituitary gland.

10. _____ One maternal change that occurs during pregnancy is an increase in blood volume of 1 to 2 L.

11. _____ Menopause occurs because of a decrease in the number of ovarian follicles.

12. _____ The greatest fetal growth occurs during the first trimester.

Matching

Match the terms in the right column with their definitions in the left column.

13. _____ Muscular area where the ureters enter the bladder

14. _____ Mediates testosterone synthesis

15. _____ Responsible for stimulating ovulation

16. _____ Secreted by the corpus luteum

17. _____ In addition to estrogen and progesterone, these hormones stimulate breast development at puberty

18. _____ Site of fertilization of the ovum by sperm

19. _____ Hormone responsible for initiating uterine contractions of labor

20. _____ Secreted by the placenta to assist in maintaining pregnancy

21. _____ The time in pregnancy when fetal movement can be felt

A. Detrusor
B. First trimester
C. Trigone
D. Uterus
E. Follicle-stimulating hormone (FSH) and luteinizing hormone (LH)
F. Fallopian tube
G. Human chorionic gonadotropin
H. Second trimester
I. Testosterone
J. LH
K. Growth hormone and prolactin
L. Oxytocin
M. Estrogen and progesterone

PATHOPHYSIOLOGY QUESTIONS
Multiple Choice

Select the one best answer to each of the following questions.

22. The most common site of urinary obstruction in male newborns and infants is:
    A. where the ureters enter the bladder wall.
    B. at the urethral valves in the distal prostatic urethra.
    C. at the urethral meatus.
    D. where the renal pelvis empties into the ureter.

23. In hypospadias the urethral meatus is located:
    A. on the ventral surface of the penis or on the perineum.
    B. on the dorsal surface of the penis near the glans.
    C. immediately anterior to the anus.
    D. midway on the shaft of the penis.

24. A persistent, painful erection is called:
    A. epispadias.
    B. paraphimosis.
    C. resistant.
    D. priapism.

25. Secondary impotence may be caused by:
    A. psychiatric problems.
    B. diabetes mellitus.
    C. vascular trauma to the penis in childhood.
    D. excessive sympathetic innervation.

26. A diagnosis of cryptorchidism increases the risk for developing:
    A. penile cancer.
    B. prostatitis.
    C. testicular cancer.
    D. impotence.

27. Testicular torsion can result in:
    A. hydrocele.
    B. testicular cancer.
    C. spermatocele.
    D. testicular death.

28. A patient presenting with a bladder infection and a swollen, red, and tender scrotum would probably be diagnosed as having:
    A. syphilis.
    B. genital herpes.
    C. epididymitis.
    D. cystocele.

29. A decrease in the diameter and force of the urinary stream, and difficulty initiating urination with dribbling at the conclusion of the void are common presenting signs and symptoms of:
    A. benign prostatic hyperplasia (BPH).
    B. prostatitis.
    C. hydrocele.
    D. urinary tract infection.

30. Amenorrhea is primarily associated with alterations in the quantity or action of:
    A. progesterone.
    B. estrogen.
    C. LH.
    D. FSH.

31. Endometrial polyps or endometrial hyperplasia are common causes of:
    A. metrorrhagia.
    B. menorrhagia.
    C. hypomenorrhea.
    D. polymenorrhea.

32. The symptoms of dysmenorrhea:
    A. are a reflection of a neurosis.
    B. are associated with an abnormal amount of menstrual bleeding.
    C. typically increase with age.
    D. can be effectively managed with drugs that inhibit prostaglandin formation.

33. Uterine prolapse, cystocele, and rectocele may all be the result of:
    A. repeated infections.
    B. chronic constipation.
    C. hormonal abnormalities.
    D. pregnancy and childbirth.

34. Pelvic inflammatory disease is managed aggressively because long-term effects can include:
    A. preterm labor.
    B. renal failure.
    C. infertility.
    D. transmission to the fetus.

35. Uterine leiomyomas (fibroids) tend to decrease after menopause because their growth appears to be dependent on:
    A. estrogen.
    B. progesterone.
    C. prolactin.
    D. testosterone.

36. Endometriosis is associated with:
    A. frequent episodes of pelvic inflammatory disease.
    B. minimal discomfort.
    C. reduced fertility rates.
    D. fluid-filled sacs attached to the endometrial wall.

37. Early stage cervical cancer may be detected by:
    A. thick gray discharge into the vagina.
    B. abnormal Pap test results.
    C. development of abnormal uterine bleeding.
    D. symptoms of urinary tract infection.

38. Fibrocystic breast disease is characterized by:
    A. an increased risk of breast cancer.
    B. benign neoplastic growths in breast tissue.
    C. a decreased ability to breast-feed offspring.
    D. breast masses that present on a cyclic basis and are tender to palpation.

39. The primary risk factor for breast cancer is:
    A. decreased estrogen.
    B. increasing age.
    C. multiparity.
    D. dietary patterns.

40. Many sexually transmitted diseases can also be contracted by:
    A. a vaginally delivered newborn of an infected mother.
    B. ingestion of contaminated food.
    C. handling of infected material.
    D. inhalation of airborne spores.

41. A patient suspected of having a sexually transmitted disease who presents with inflammation of the urethra, uterine cervix, and/or signs and symptoms of pelvic inflammatory disease most likely is infected with:
    A. *Neisseria gonorrhoeae.*
    B. *Treponema pallidum.*
    C. Herpes virus.
    D. *Haemophilus ducreyi.*

42. The sexually transmitted disease that begins with formation of a painless ulcer (called a chancre) and later progresses to a systemic form is:
    A. herpes.
    B. chlamydial infection.
    C. syphilis.
    D. hepatitis B.

43. Herpes virus type 2 may remain in the body in a latent form. Exacerbations of the disease may be triggered by:
    A. reinfection.
    B. sexual intercourse.
    C. temperature extremes.
    D. emotional stress.

44. Which of the following statements about genital warts *(Condylomata acuminata)* is false?
    A. They are highly contagious.
    B. They are rarely visible because the growths develop deep in tissues.
    C. They are due to infection with a type of human papilloma virus.
    D. They have an incubation period averaging 4 months.

Fill in the Blank

Fill in the following blanks with the appropriate word or words.

45. Differentiation of primitive gonadal tissues into ovaries and testes begins at the _____ week of gestation.

46. Epididymitis is most frequently caused by _____.

47. The organism most commonly responsible for prostatitis is _____.

48. The _____ is the inner layer of uterine tissue that proliferates and is then sloughed during menstruation.

49. The decline in estrogen associated with menopause results in _____, which increases a woman's risk for fractures.

50. Protrusion of the bladder wall into the vagina is called a _____ and is most often due to _____.

51. Pregnancy-induced hypertension can be screened for by monitoring blood pressure and testing the urine for _____.

52. Transient nausea is most common in the _____ trimester of pregnancy.

53. Transmission of *Chlamydia* during childbirth can result in an infection of the _____ of the newborn.

Case Studies

I.L. is a healthy 28-year-old woman, pregnant with her first child. A nursing student is visiting her and her husband. The student's primary responsibility is to identify learning needs and design teaching plans to address those needs. I.L. and her husband are fascinated with the changes in her body and learning about the development of the fetus.

54. "I understand that the placenta is responsible for bringing oxygen and nutrients to the fetus, but does it serve any other function?" asks I.L. The student would be correct in responding:
    A. "Yes, it also secretes hormones that increase the size of the uterus and make structures more elastic for delivery."
    B. "No, that is the only function that the placenta performs."
    C. "Yes, it stabilizes the embryo when it is very small so that it cannot leave the uterus."
    D. "Yes, it secretes hormones that maintain the mother's health during pregnancy."

55. In response to I.L.'s question about weight gain during pregnancy, the student would be correct in basing a reply on the fact that:
    A. most of the weight gain occurs in the second and third trimesters.
    B. the average weight gain in pregnancy is 35 pounds.
    C. the weight of the fetus constitutes most of the total weight gain.
    D. most of the weight gained, beyond the weight of the fetus, is attributable to edema fluid.

56. The student tells I.L. that all of the following changes in her body would be normal except:
    A. breasts doubling in size.
    B. an increase in respiratory rate.
    C. slight elevation in temperature.
    D. swelling of the face, especially around the eyes.

57. The primary nutrient a pregnant woman needs, since stored levels are not sufficient to meet the maternal and fetal needs, is:
    A. calcium.
    B. vitamin C.
    C. iron.
    D. magnesium.

F.R. is 47 years old and has come to see her physician for her annual physical. During their conversation, F.R. describes a menstrual pattern that has been irregular over the past few months. She wonders if she might be experiencing menopause.

58. Additional signs or symptoms of menopause may include:
    A. increased frequency of urination.
    B. sudden sensations of warmth of the neck and face.
    C. clear, thick discharge from the vagina.
    D. muscle aches.

59. The underlying cause of menopause is:
    A. sealing of the cervix.
    B. structural changes in the uterus.
    C. estrogen deficiency.
    D. progesterone excess.

60. The changes associated with perimenopause and menopause increase the risk for:
    A. lung diseases such as asthma.
    B. osteoporosis.
    C. autoimmune diseases.
    D. type 2 diabetes.

A 19-year-old female student comes to the Student Health Center complaining of painful urination, suspicious of a urinary tract infection. A laboratory analysis report indicates a gonococcal infection.

61. In women, gonorrhea:
    A. is uncommon.
    B. has no effect on later reproduction.
    C. usually has no symptoms.
    D. always coexists with *Chlamydia trachomatis* infection.

62. In men, gonorrhea:
    A. usually has no symptoms.
    B. frequently causes urinary tract infection.
    C. may cause inflammation of the Bartholin glands.
    D. may result in epididymitis.

63. In patients with symptomatic gonorrhea, the infection may cause inflammation of the:
    A. pharynx.
    B. retina.
    C. joints.
    D. heart valves.

B.H. is a 53-year-old woman who discovered a lump in her breast while performing breast self-examination. Upon seeing her physician and having a mammogram and biopsy, she is convinced that she has a carcinoma of the breast.

64. A major difference found on breast self-examination between malignant and benign growths in the breast is that malignant growths are:
   A. smaller.
   B. nontender.
   C. somewhat movable.
   D. softer to the touch.

65. A review of B.H.'s history reveals which of the following as a significant risk factor for breast cancer?
   A. Onset of menses at age 13 and menopause at age 50
   B. A mother with breast cancer
   C. History of fibrocystic breast disease
   D. A diet averaging 20% fat

66. The most common location for malignant tumors of the breast is the:
   A. nipple area.
   B. inner aspect, near the sternum.
   C. lower surface.
   D. upper, outer quadrant.

67. Prognosis for breast cancer is most contingent on:
   A. size of the tumor.
   B. location of the tumor in the breast.
   C. age of the woman.
   D. degree of lymph node involvement.

Sixty-five-year-old D.E. comes to see his physician with complaints of difficulty initiating his urinary stream, and dribbling after voiding. He has postponed this doctor's appointment out of fear that he might have prostate cancer. But recently, he began to have frequency, urgency and some dysuria, so he followed through with the appointment; he's still very worried. His physician draws blood for a serum prostate-specific antigen.

68. A significantly elevated level of prostate-specific antigen is indicative of:
   A. prostate cancer.
   B. BPH.
   C. either prostate cancer or BPH.
   D. the absence of any pathologic process, as low levels indicate disease.

69. The symptoms of urinary tract infection in the presence of an enlarged, painless prostate gland are most characteristic of:
   A. prostate cancer.
   B. prostatitis.
   C. BPH.
   D. any condition affecting the prostate gland.

70. The primary etiologic factor associated with the development of BPH appears to be:
   A. recurrent infection.
   B. a viral infection elsewhere in the body.
   C. increasing age of the male endocrine system.
   D. urinary retention.

ANATOMY REVIEW
Matching

1. b, e, h, d, c, a, g, f
2. a, f, g, d, e, c, b

NORMAL ANATOMY
AND PHYSIOLOGY REVIEW
True/False

3. T
4. F
5. F
6. F
7. T
8. F
9. T
10. T
11. T
12. F

Matching

13. C
14. J
15. E
16. M
17. K
18. F
19. L
20. G
21. H

PATHOPHYSIOLOGY QUESTIONS
Multiple Choice

22. B
23. A
24. D
25. B
26. C
27. D
28. C
29. A
30. B
31. B

32. D
33. D
34. C
35. A
36. C
37. B
38. D
39. B
40. A
41. A
42. C
43. D
44. B

Fill in the Blank

45. seventh
46. infection
47. *E. coli*
48. endometrium
49. osteoporosis
50. cystocele; childbirth
51. protein
52. first
53. eyes

Case Studies

54. A
55. A
56. D
57. C
58. B
59. C
60. B
61. C
62. D
63. A
64. B
65. B
66. D
67. D
68. A
69. C
70. C

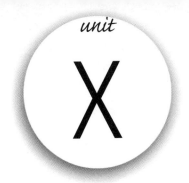

Gastrointestinal Function

Chapters 35 to 38

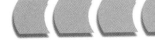

ANATOMY REVIEW
Matching
1. Match each lettered item in the figure with one of the following anatomic terms:

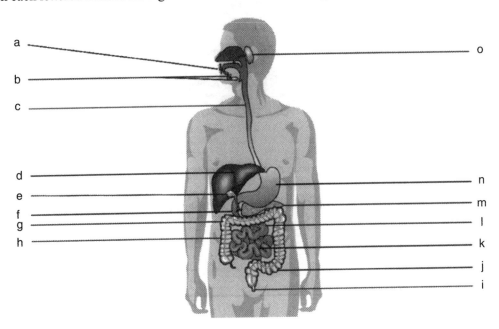

_____	Anus	_____	Descending colon
_____	Liver	_____	Parotid glands
_____	Ascending colon	_____	Duodenum
_____	Mouth	_____	Pancreas
_____	Esophagus	_____	Ileum
_____	Salivary glands	_____	Transverse colon
_____	Gallbladder	_____	Jejunum
_____	Stomach		

2. Match each lettered item in the figure with one of the following anatomic terms:

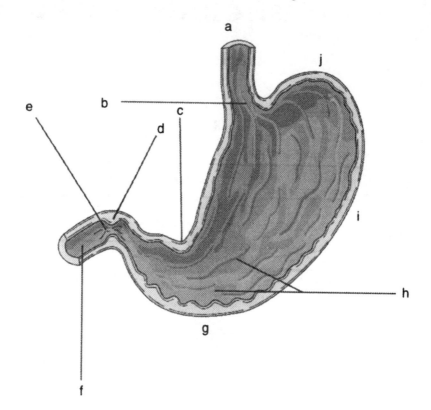

_____ Angular notch

_____ Esophagus

_____ Antrum

_____ Fundus

_____ Body

_____ Pyloric sphincter

_____ Cardia

_____ Pylorus

_____ Duodenum

_____ Rugae

NORMAL ANATOMY AND PHYSIOLOGY REVIEW
True/False

Indicate whether the following statements regarding the anatomy and physiology of the gastrointestinal system are true (T) or false (F).

3. _____ The intrinsic nervous system of the gastrointestinal tract has a greater role in the control of its functions than does the autonomic nervous system.

4. _____ Secretion of bile from the gallbladder is stimulated by gastrin release into the stomach.

5. _____ If the contents of the duodenum are acidic or hypertonic, gastric emptying may be slowed.

6. _____ Parasympathetic stimulation of the large bowel produces increased motility.

7. _____ Propulsion of gastrointestinal contents is primarily regulated by the autonomic nervous system.

8. _____ The vomiting center is located in the central nervous system.

9. _____ Parietal cells of the stomach secrete pepsinogen, which is activated to pepsin in the presence of intrinsic factor.

10. _____ Digestion of carbohydrates is initiated by release of amylase released into the duodenum by the pancreas.

11. _____ No digestion of dietary fats occurs until they reach the small intestine.

12. _____ The primary site of nutrient and water absorption is the small intestine.

13. _____ Unlike fat or carbohydrate digestion, protein digestion begins in the stomach.

14. _____ Fat emulsification involves the enzymatic breakdown of large lipid molecules by bile.

15. _____ Water absorption from the gastrointestinal tract occurs via active transport systems.

16. _____ The lower esophageal sphincter (LES) will not release food into the stomach until it has been fully processed by salivary digestive enzymes.

17. _____ Babies younger than 3 to 4 months must be fed only liquids because their enzyme systems are too immature to break down solid foods.

18. _____ The secretory and absorptive functions of the intestine are not fully mature for the first 2 years of life.

19. _____ Decreased intake in the elderly is most commonly a result of their reduced basal metabolic rate.

20. _____ Intestinal transit time increases with age, increasing the risk for constipation in the elderly.

PATHOPHYSIOLOGY QUESTIONS
Compare/Contrast

Compare and contrast ulcerative colitis and Crohn disease by filling in "yes" or "no" in the appropriate column.

Characteristic	Ulcerative Colitis	Crohn Disease
Abscess formation		
Bloody diarrhea		
Fistula formation		
Rectal bleeding		
Mucosal layer involvement		
Transmural involvement		

Fill in the Blank

Fill in the blanks with the appropriate word or words.

21. A common cause of constipation is a _____ _____ diet.

22. In Western countries, acute gastritis is most commonly associated with the overuse of _____, _____, and _____.

23. _____ ulcers usually cause pain when the stomach is empty or shortly after eating, whereas _____ ulcers cause pain 2 to 3 hours after eating.

24. Conditions that may result in mechanical bowel obstruction include _____, which is a twisted bowel, and _____, in which the bowel telescopes upon itself.

25. An acquired bowel disease that may develop at any age, _____ is most often caused by prolonged constipation.

Multiple Choice

Select the one best answer to each of the following questions.

26. All of the following may result in dysphagia except:
     A. altered neuromuscular ability to coordinate movement of material to the esophagus.
     B. impaired relaxation of the LES.
     C. decreased peristalsis of the distal portion of the esophagus.
     D. pyrosis.

27. Abdominal pain that manifests as visceral pain is characterized by:
     A. sensations at a distant site, along the same dermatome route as the original location.
     B. being extremely sharp and well localized.
     C. diaphragmatic or peritoneal involvement.
     D. being diffuse and poorly localized, with a cramping or burning sensation.

28. The diarrhea seen with inflammatory bowel disease is primarily an example of:
    A. osmotic diarrhea.
    B. secretory diarrhea.
    C. exudative diarrhea.
    D. diarrhea due to increased motility.

29. A common cause of stomatitis seen in immunosuppressed patients is:
    A. *Candida albicans*.
    B. vitamin deficiency.
    C. exposure to chemical irritants.
    D. gastroesophageal reflux.

30. Mallory-Weiss syndrome usually is caused by:
    A. hiatal hernia.
    B. overdosage with acetaminophen.
    C. cirrhosis.
    D. severe vomiting episode.

31. Risk factors for gastroesophageal reflux include:
    A. hiatal hernia.
    B. constipation.
    C. esophagitis.
    D. decreased gastric acidity.

32. *Helicobacter pylori* infection has been implicated in all of the following except:
    A. chronic gastritis.
    B. gastric cancer.
    C. peptic ulcer disease (PUD).
    D. acute gastritis.

33. Common manifestations of PUD include:
    A. diarrhea.
    B. burning epigastric pain.
    C. hematemesis.
    D. frank blood in the stool.

34. A patient with PUD should be encouraged to avoid:
    A. spicy foods.
    B. aspirin and nonsteroidal antiinflammatory drugs (NSAIDs).
    C. excessive intake of liquids.
    D. lying down immediately after eating.

35. A major predisposing factor to the development of pseudomembranous enterocolitis is:
    A. history of inflammatory bowel disease.
    B. intestinal hypoxia.
    C. antibiotic therapy.
    D. contaminated foods.

36. The primary life-threatening complication of appendicitis is:
    A. peritonitis.
    B. dehydration.
    C. cardiac arrest.
    D. abscess formation.

37. Which of the following is a true statement regarding diverticular disease?
    A. It can occur anywhere in the small or large intestine.
    B. It most frequently affects young adults.
    C. If diverticuli become inflamed, intestinal obstruction may result.
    D. The condition is most common among societies where the diet is high in cellulose.

38. All of the following could result in a mechanical bowel obstruction except:
    A. volvulus.
    B. intussusception.
    C. adhesions.
    D. narcotic analgesic administration.

39. The manifestations of bowel obstruction are primarily related to:
    A. decreased absorption of nutrients.
    B. accumulation of fluid and gas proximal to the obstruction.
    C. edema impairing biliary secretion.
    D. death of intestinal bacteria.

40. A congenital condition of the colon in which there are insufficient autonomic ganglia in the bowel resulting in contraction but inadequate relaxation to move the fecal mass forward efficiently is called:
    A. short-bowel syndrome.
    B. celiac disease.
    C. irritable bowel syndrome.
    D. Hirschsprung disease.

41. All malabsorptive conditions:
    A. are due to mucosal dysfunction.
    B. are due to enzymatic dysfunction.
    C. affect the colon.
    D. affect the small intestine.

42. Carcinoma of the stomach is:
    A. slow growing and therefore highly curable with early diagnosis.
    B. associated with precancerous polyps.
    C. highly correlated with *H. pylori* infection.
    D. primarily managed with chemotherapy.

43. Warning signs for colon cancer include:
    A. blood in the stool.
    B. epigastric pain.
    C. nausea or vomiting after meals.
    D. loss of appetite.

44. Risk factors for gallstone formation include all of the following except:
    A. female gender.
    B. cystic fibrosis.
    C. gastritis.
    D. obesity.

45. Patients with acute pancreatitis are closely monitored for the development of the potentially lethal complication of:
    A. pancreatic rupture.
    B. circulatory shock.
    C. cardiac dysrhythmias.
    D. stroke.

46. Like acute pancreatitis, the development of chronic pancreatitis is frequently associated with:
    A. biliary disease.
    B. diabetes.
    C. alcohol abuse.
    D. malnutrition.

47. Hepatocellular failure produces all of the following except:
    A. jaundice.
    B. edema.
    C. bleeding tendencies.
    D. decrease of all water-soluble vitamins.

48. An elevation in conjugated bilirubin would be seen in all of the following except:
    A. massive hemolysis.
    B. neonates.
    C. viral hepatitis.
    D. mechanical obstruction of the colon.

49. Impaired blood flow through the liver results in portal hypertension. This may produce:
    A. osteomalacia.
    B. esophageal varices.
    C. impaired activation of vitamin D.
    D. hepatic coma.

50. The encephalopathy seen with liver failure is associated with the inability of the liver to:
    A. conjugate bilirubin for excretion.
    B. synthesize albumin to maintain oncotic pressure.
    C. metabolize hormones, especially aldosterone and estrogen.
    D. convert ammonia to urea for excretion.

51. Acute renal failure due to liver failure (hepatorenal syndrome) is due to:
    A. diminished intrarenal blood flow.
    B. obstruction of the ureters as they exit the renal pelvis.
    C. accumulation of unmetabolized waste in the renal tubules.
    D. pressure on the renal arteries by ascitic fluid.

52. Hepatitis A:
    A. is spread by contact with contaminated body fluids, such as blood or wound drainage.
    B. has an incubation period of up to 4 months.
    C. can be prevented through immunization.
    D. typically leaves the patient with permanently impaired liver function.

53. Hepatitis B and hepatitis C share a similar:
    A. incubation period.
    B. prophylactic vaccine.
    C. incidence of progression to chronic liver disease.
    D. mode of transmission.

54. Chronic hepatitis, regardless of the specific disease, is characterized by:
    A. continuing liver inflammation for 6 months or longer following the initial insult.
    B. a viral etiology.
    C. progression to liver cancer or cirrhosis.
    D. diffuse scarring and fibrosis of the liver.

55. A common cause of asymptomatically abnormal liver laboratory tests is:
    A. hepatitis.
    B. fatty liver.
    C. gallbladder disease.
    D. toxic liver disorders.

56. The underlying pathologic mechanism of hemochromatosis is:
    A. excessive absorption of dietary iron.
    B. excessive accumulation of dietary copper.
    C. formation of excessive amounts of hemoglobin.
    D. formation of excessive amounts of activated vitamin D.

57. Children or adults consuming excessive amounts of acetaminophen are at risk for:
    A. cirrhosis.
    B. liver necrosis.
    C. increased bleeding in the liver.
    D. impaired gastrointestinal functioning.

58. Cancer of the liver is:
    A. a risk associated with hepatitis A.
    B. rarely associated with cirrhosis.
    C. usually due to metastasis from another site.
    D. most often managed by surgical resection.

59. Liver abscess:
    A. may be due to infection by *H. pylori*.
    B. requires surgical intervention.
    C. should be considered in patients with fever and right upper quadrant pain.
    D. frequently recurs.

60. Trauma to the liver:
    A. can result in significant blood loss.
    B. is only a concern with abdominal trauma.
    C. rarely requires surgical intervention.
    D. is accompanied by signs and symptoms of systemic infection.

Case Studies

T.W. is a 52-year-old man who has developed cirrhosis secondary to repeated, prolonged exposure to alcohol. He has most recently been hospitalized because of an upper gastrointestinal bleed due to the rupture of esophageal varices.

61. T.W.'s skin and the sclera of his eyes have a yellowish cast. The nurse knows that this jaundice is due to:
    A. release of excessive amounts of bilirubin from red blood cells.
    B. increased quantities of conjugated bilirubin.
    C. excessive contraction of the sphincter of Oddi.
    D. increased quantities of unconjugated bilirubin.

62. The development of esophageal varices in cirrhosis is related to:
    A. hepatic fibrosis causing increased resistance to portal circulation.
    B. impairment of venous drainage from the thorax to the liver.
    C. increased vascular volume due to hepatorenal failure.
    D. pressure increases due to prolonged vomiting.

63. Signs and symptoms of upper gastrointestinal hemorrhage include:
    A. rapid decrease in hematocrit.
    B. confusion, disorientation, and coma.
    C. hematemesis.
    D. abdominal distention.

64. Interventions that are used in the management of esophageal varices by decreasing portal hypertension include:
    A. blood transfusions.
    B. endoscopic sclerosis.
    C. β-blockers or nitroglycerin.
    D. balloon tamponade.

65. Ruptured esophageal varices can produce profound hemorrhage. An additional pathologic feature of cirrhosis that contributes to hemorrhage is:
    A. hypoalbuminemia.
    B. impaired protein metabolism, which decreases production of clotting factors.
    C. altered production of lipoproteins.
    D. impaired glycogenesis and glycogenolysis.

C.D. comes to the clinic complaining of a long-lasting gastrointestinal flu. He tells the nurse that he became ill about a month after returning from a visit with friends in another state. Further investigation determines that one of C.D.'s friends has similar symptoms. Laboratory studies reveal a slight increase in aspartate aminotransferase (AST) levels, a total bilirubin of 1.5 mg/dl, and positive anti-hepatitis A virus IgM.

66. These laboratory tests are indicative of:
    A. immunity to hepatitis A.
    B. past infection with hepatitis A.
    C. active infection with hepatitis A.
    D. exposure but no infection with hepatitis A.

67. Physical signs and symptoms of hepatitis include all of the following except:
    A. anorexia.
    B. low-grade fever.
    C. acute left upper quadrant abdominal pain.
    D. nausea.

68. The most common means of contracting hepatitis A is:
    A. poor personal hygiene.
    B. sexual intercourse.
    C. contaminated needles or blood transfusion.
    D. ingestion of contaminated food or water.

D.D. is a 43-year-old woman who comes into the emergency room complaining of acute abdominal pain. She states that the pain came on after dinner at an "all-you-can-eat" buffet and has been increasing steadily. The pain is located in her right upper quadrant and is "boring" into her back. She says she feels "gassy" and bloated.

69. The emergency department physician suspects cholecystitis and orders:
    A. a complete blood count.
    B. an abdominal x-ray.
    C. a total, conjugated, and unconjugated bilirubin level.
    D. an abdominal ultrasound.

70. The cause of cholecystitis usually is:
    A. a viral infection.
    B. hepatocellular failure.
    C. biliary obstruction by gallstones.
    D. biliary atresia.

71. The advantage of cholecystectomy over chemical dissolution and lithotripsy is:
    A. decreased cost.
    B. no recurrence of the cholecystitis.
    C. less risk of diarrhea.
    D. fewer dietary alterations.

72. The principal complication of unmanaged cholecystitis is:
    A. rupture of the gallbladder.
    B. sepsis.
    C. hemorrhage.
    D. inability to digest fats.

73. The most common point of biliary obstruction by cholelithiasis is:
    A. the common bile duct.
    B. the cystic duct.
    C. the duodenal papilla.
    D. the sphincter of Oddi.

M.N. has rheumatoid arthritis and takes high doses of aspirin to control his pain and maintain function. He has had problems with gastritis from the aspirin, but it seemed to be relieved when he switched to enteric-coated aspirin and started taking it with food. Now, however, it seems to be worse. He came to the clinic complaining of increasing abdominal distress, and a gastric ulcer was diagnosed.

74. Aspirin and NSAIDs are causative factors for the development of PUD because they:
    A. increase acid secretion.
    B. allow proliferation of *H. pylori*.
    C. damage the mucosal barrier.
    D. alter platelet aggregation.

75. Although by themselves they are not the cause of PUD, all of the following can contribute to the condition except:
    A. smoking.
    B. caffeine.
    C. alcohol.
    D. estrogen.

76. M.N.'s therapy for his rheumatoid arthritis is changed. Another intervention that will contribute to the healing of his peptic ulcers is:
    A. steroid administration.
    B. blocking or neutralizing of acid secretion.
    C. surgical removal of the ulcer.
    D. intravenous nutritional support.

77. Pepsin, a proteolytic enzyme found in the gastrointestinal tract, is converted from its precursor form, pepsinogen, in the presence of:
    A. HCO_3^- secretions from the pancreas delivered to the duodenum.
    B. HCl secretions in the stomach.
    C. *H. pylori* bacteria, in residence in the epithelial wall.
    D. gastrin secretions in the stomach.

A.G. is a 32-year-old accountant who has been dealing with Crohn disease since her early twenties. She has had one bowel resection, which provided some improvement of symptoms for a few years. She comes to the clinic for a routine evaluation of her therapeutic regimen.

78. Crohn disease differs pathologically from ulcerative colitis in that ulcerative colitis:
    A. affects only the mucosal layer of the bowel.
    B. involves the small and large bowel.
    C. produces a greater risk for malabsorption of nutrients.
    D. may progress to development of fistulas in adjacent organs.

79. Management of both Crohn disease and ulcerative colitis focuses on:
    A. decreasing inflammation with drug therapy.
    B. reducing intake of foods that are high in fiber.
    C. limiting fluid intake during episodes of diarrhea.
    D. antibiotic therapy to eliminate the causative organisms.

80. Crohn disease and ulcerative colitis both:
    A. typically develop in young adulthood.
    B. produce stool that is watery, and filled with mucus and pus.
    C. have remissions with full recovery of pathologic changes in the bowel.
    D. cause adhesions in the bowel.

ANATOMY REVIEW
Matching

1. i, d, h, a, c, b, e, n, j, o, f, m, k, g, l
2. c, a, g, j, i, d, b, e, f, h

NORMAL ANATOMY
AND PHYSIOLOGY REVIEW
True/False

3. T
4. F
5. T
6. T
7. F
8. T
9. F
10. F
11. T
12. T
13. T
14. F
15. F
16. F
17. F
18. T
19. F
20. T

PATHOPHYSIOLOGY QUESTIONS
Compare/Contrast

Characteristic	Ulcerative Colitis	Crohn Disease
Abscess formation	Yes	Yes
Bloody diarrhea	Yes	Yes
Fistula formation	No	Yes
Rectal bleeding	Yes	No
Mucosal layer involvement	Yes	Yes
Transmural involvement	No	Yes

Fill in the Blank

21. low fiber
22. NSAIDs, alcohol, tobacco
23. gastric, duodenal
24. volvulus, intussusception
25. megacolon

Multiple Choice

26. D
27. D
28. C
29. A
30. D
31. A
32. D
33. B
34. B
35. C
36. A
37. C
38. D
39. B
40. D
41. D
42. C
43. A
44. C
45. B
46. C
47. D
48. D
49. B
50. D
51. A
52. C
53. D
54. A

55. B
56. A
57. B
58. C
59. C
60. A

Case Studies

61. D
62. A
63. C
64. C
65. B
66. C

67. C
68. D
69. D
70. C
71. B
72. A
73. B
74. C
75. D
76. B
77. B
78. A
79. A
80. A

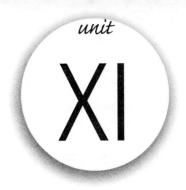

unit XI

Endocrine Function, Metabolism, and Nutrition

Chapters 39 to 42

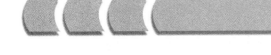

NORMAL ANATOMY AND PHYSIOLOGY REVIEW
Matching

Match the terms in the right column with their definitions in the left column. Not all terms are defined.

1. _____ Prolonged exposure to high levels of a hormone can produce this response by the hormone receptors.

2. _____ Water-soluble hormones produce their effect upon binding to cell membrane receptors by activating these.

3. _____ "Hormone-like" chemicals secreted by one cell that affect adjacent cells.

4. _____ Hormones synthesized here travel via nerve axons to the posterior pituitary for release.

5. _____ Lipid-soluble hormones, like thyroid hormone, must be attached to these to be transported in the blood.

6. _____ Hormones that are lipid soluble and are derived from cholesterol are known as _____.

7. _____ Cortisol is an example of a hormone whose release varies over a 24-hour period called a _____ pattern.

8. _____ This circulating thyroid hormone must be converted to its active form to be biologically active.

9. _____ Releasing hormones from the hypothalamus, secreted into the blood stream, stimulate hormone secretion from the

_____.

10. _____ The primary mechanism by which hormone levels in the blood are controlled.

A. Steroids
B. Hypothalamus
C. Trophic hormone
D. Down-regulation
E. Paracrine
F. Up-regulation
G. Proteins
H. Autocrine
I. Second messengers
J. Lower
K. Anterior pituitary
L. Circadian
M. T_3
N. Positive feedback
O. T_4
P. Negative feedback

True/False

Indicate whether the following statements regarding the anatomy and physiology of the endocrine system are true (T) or false (F).

11. _____ Release of the primary mineralocorticoid, aldosterone, is controlled by adrenocorticotropic hormone from the anterior pituitary.

12. _____ Neurons do not require the presence of insulin to transport glucose.

13. _____ Hormone resistance can be identified when circulating levels of the hormone are normal or elevated but target organ function is deficient.

14. _____ Hormones are easily excreted from the body and do not require metabolism.

15. _____ "Receptor specificity" means that the cells of a given tissue will respond only to hormones for which it has receptors.

16. _____ Receptor activation occurs with a hormone antagonist.

17. _____ As the proportion of body fat increases with aging, lipid metabolism may be affected.

18. _____ Pharmacologic levels of hormones are higher than physiologic levels.

19. _____ Primary endocrine disease is differentiated from secondary endocrine disease in that the problem is with the target glands.

20. _____ A major difference between starvation and physiologic stress is that in starvation the body tries to conserve lean body mass (muscle/protein).

PATHOPHYSIOLOGY QUESTIONS
Fill in the Blank

Fill in the blanks with the appropriate word or words.

21. Drug therapy for type _____ diabetes mellitus is the replacement of insulin, which is absent from the body.

22. The classic clinical manifestations of diabetes mellitus are _____, _____, _____, and _____ _____.

23. An excess of growth hormone in adults is called _____, whereas in childhood it results in _____ _____.

24. The primary intervention for syndrome of inappropriate antidiuretic hormone secretion (SIADH) is the restriction of _____ intake.

25. Manifestations of hyperparathyroidism and hypoparathyroidism are related to excessive or insufficient amounts of _____.

26. Endocrine diseases characterized as hyporesponsive are clinically similar to hyposecretion of hormones, but are due to _____ _____.

27. In primary hypothyroidism, the circulating level of thyroid-stimulating hormone (TSH) will be
_____.

28. A unique feature of Graves disease is the protrusion of the eyeballs, called _____.

29. The most common cause of hypoparathyroidism is _____ in the area where the glands are
located.

30. The primary deleterious effects of immobility are _____ _____ and _____
_____.

Multiple Choice

Select the one best answer to each of the following questions.

31. Children with a deficiency in growth hormone may demonstrate which of the following manifestations?
    A. Early onset of puberty
    B. Bone overgrowth producing bony tumors
    C. Early loss of primary dentition
    D. Decreased height for chronological age

32. All of the following hormones increase blood glucose levels except:
    A. cortisol.
    B. oxytocin.
    C. growth hormone.
    D. norepinephrine.

33. Diabetes insipidus is characterized by:
    A. hypernatremia.
    B. neurologic symptoms associated with swelling of brain cells.
    C. weight gain.
    D. increased urine specific gravity.

34. Causes of acquired hypothyroidism include all of the following except:
    A. goitrogenic foods.
    B. Hashimoto thyroiditis.
    C. cretinism.
    D. insufficient iodine intake.

35. Hypothyroidism manifestations include:
    A. heat intolerance.
    B. moist, warm skin.
    C. nonpitting edema.
    D. insomnia.

36. In Graves disease:
    A. circulating levels of thyroid hormones are decreased.
    B. an autoimmune process affects TSH receptors.
    C. metabolic rate is slowed.
    D. too much thyroid replacement therapy has been administered.

37. Congenital hypothyroidism that is not managed is a serious concern because of the risk for:
    A. mental retardation.
    B. respiratory distress.
    C. heart failure.
    D. seizures.

38. Parathyroid hormone exerts control over serum calcium maintenance by affecting all of the following except:
    A. osteoclastic/osteoblastic activity.
    B. renal tubular reabsorption of calcium.
    C. renal activation of vitamin D and gastrointestinal absorption of dietary calcium.
    D. mineralization of the teeth.

39. A patient with hyperparathyroidism would be likely to present with:
    A. elevated calcitonin levels.
    B. increased deep tendon reflexes.
    C. numbness and tingling of fingers or toes.
    D. kidney stones.

40. A potentially life-threatening finding in hypoparathyroidism is:
    A. laryngospasm.
    B. Trousseau sign.
    C. Chvostek sign.
    D. heart failure.

41. Cortisol, the body's primary glucocorticoid:
    A. is released from the anterior pituitary.
    B. increases glycogenesis.
    C. is a catabolic hormone.
    D. enhances the inflammatory response.

42. Findings associated with primary adrenal insufficiency/Addison disease include:
    A. fluid retention.
    B. hypokalemia.
    C. hyperglycemia.
    D. hyponatremia.

43. Classic manifestations seen with Cushing syndrome include all of the following except:
    A. bruising due to capillary fragility.
    B. hypertrophy of muscle tissue.
    C. increased susceptibility to infections.
    D. pathologic fractures.

44. Aldosterone promotes reabsorption of sodium and water, as well as excretion of potassium by the kidneys. What other hormone also produces these effects?
    A. Antidiuretic hormone
    B. Cortisol
    C. Thyroid hormone
    D. Parathyroid hormone

45. Pheochromocytoma is a rare, life-threatening disease characterized by:
    A. profound hypertension.
    B. circulatory collapse from dehydration.
    C. respiratory arrest.
    D. total absence of a stress response.

46. Type 1 diabetes mellitus differs from type 2 in that:
    A. the onset is usually in middle or later adulthood.
    B. it is associated with insulin resistance.
    C. it is the most common form of diabetes.
    D. there is an absolute deficiency of insulin production.

47. Ketoacidosis is uncommon in type 2 diabetes because:
    A. dehydration is less severe.
    B. endogenous insulin prevents lipolysis and production of ketone bodies.
    C. metabolic acidosis does not occur.
    D. liver breakdown of stored glycogen to glucose does not produce fatty acids.

48. Women who develop gestational diabetes:
    A. will probably remain diabetic following delivery of their babies.
    B. give birth to babies with low birth weights who are hyperglycemic.
    C. are primarily treated with any of the available oral agents.
    D. are likely to experience it with subsequent pregnancies.

49. Microvascular complications occurring with chronic hyperglycemia in diabetes mellitus, such as retinopathy and nephropathy, are associated with:
    A. thickening of capillary basement membranes.
    B. atrophy of vascular tissues.
    C. slowed perfusion due to the hyperosmolar state.
    D. impaired oxygen binding to hemoglobin.

50. A sign of early diabetic nephropathy is:
    A. anuria.
    B. glycosuria.
    C. hypertension.
    D. microalbuminuria.

51. Neuropathy of autonomic and sensory nerves seen in diabetes mellitus is associated with:
    A. decreased myoinositol in cell membranes of peripheral nerves.
    B. increased formation of atherosclerotic plaques.
    C. decreased myelination.
    D. increased distances between nodes of Ranvier.

52. Dietary recommendations for management of diabetes mellitus include:
    A. protein intake constituting 30% of the daily caloric intake.
    B. polyunsaturated fat intake of 20% of the daily caloric intake.
    C. low to moderate alcohol intake, always accompanied by food.
    D. 50% of the daily caloric intake distributed between fats and carbohydrates.

53. Exercise for the patient with type 2 diabetes may result in:
    A. improved renal function.
    B. decreased insulin resistance.
    C. decreased risk of eating disorder development.
    D. increased low-density lipid levels.

54. Signs or symptoms of hypoglycemia include all of the following except:
    A. pallor.
    B. tremors.
    C. fever.
    D. altered consciousness.

55. Which of the following is true regarding complications of diabetes in children?
    A. Neuropathies are common and develop early in the disease.
    B. Diabetic ketoacidosis rarely occurs.
    C. Dehydration is a major concern when hyperglycemia is severe.
    D. Manifestations of hypoglycemia in very young children are identical to those seen in adults.

56. In the elderly population, complications of diabetes and aging increase the risk for the development of:
    A. hyperglycemia.
    B. hypoglycemia.
    C. diabetic ketoacidosis.
    D. heart disease.

57. Biochemical tests indicative of either a poor intake of protein or protein utilization by the liver are:
    A. low transferrin, albumin, and prealbumin levels.
    B. elevated blood urea nitrogen (BUN) and creatinine levels.
    C. decreased red blood cell and hemoglobin levels.
    D. increased hematocrit and white blood cell count.

58. During the immediate phase of acute physiologic stress, glucose utilization is impaired. Provision of an excessive amount of carbohydrates at this time may result in:
    A. hypoglycemia.
    B. excessive production of carbon dioxide.
    C. increased production of heat in the body.
    D. hyperlipidemia.

59. A significant complication that malnourished patients may develop when feeding is resumed is:
    A. heart failure.
    B. infections.
    C. respiratory failure.
    D. muscle spasms.

60. Patients who are malnourished prior to surgery are at increased risk for:
    A. impaired gastrointestinal motility.
    B. increased basal metabolic rate.
    C. poor wound healing.
    D. muscle atrophy.

Case Studies

Eight-year-old W.E. has been brought to the doctor's office by his parents. Over the past few days, he has been weak, complaining of being very thirsty and hungry. They have noticed he urinates more frequently. Laboratory tests in combination with this history confirm the diagnosis of type 1 diabetes mellitus.

61. The polyuria associated with diabetes is due to:
    A. the polydipsia.
    B. the osmotic effects of glycosuria.
    C. increased protein catabolism.
    D. the loss of electrolytes.

62. Excessive ketone production will produce what laboratory finding?
    A. Increased partial pressure of carbon dioxide
    B. Decreased hematocrit
    C. Decreased pH
    D. Increased BUN

63. The rapid, deep respirations associated with ketoacidosis (Kussmaul respirations) are the result of the body's attempt to:
    A. compensate for metabolic acidosis.
    B. combat hypoxemia.
    C. increase the partial pressure of oxygen.
    D. improve the level of consciousness.

64. Since W.E. has type 1 diabetes, insulin therapy will be required. At his age, W.E. can be taught to monitor his blood sugar and administer his own insulin injections with supervision. All of the following statements regarding pediatric considerations in the administration of insulin and monitoring blood glucose levels are true except:
    A. Adequate treatment is essential to ensure normal growth and maturation.
    B. As with adults, the abdomen is the preferred site for injections.
    C. An intensive regimen of at least three injections per day helps to avoid chronic complications.
    D. If doses are very small, a diluent may be needed to ensure adequate drug delivery.

65. The best laboratory test to monitor how well W.E.'s blood sugar levels are being managed over time is:
    A. testing for glucose in the urine.
    B. fasting blood glucose level.
    C. spot checking blood glucose level.
    D. glycosylated hemoglobin.

N.M., a 45-year-old woman, was diagnosed with hypothyroidism 10 years ago. Her condition has been effectively managed with thyroid replacement therapy.

66. The most likely cause of N.M.'s hypothyroidism would be a history of:
    A. cretinism.
    B. thyroid dysgenesis.
    C. Hashimoto thyroiditis.
    D. Graves disease.

67. Laboratory results that would indicate a primary cause of hypothyroidism would be decreased T_4 and:
    A. increased TSH.
    B. decreased TSH.
    C. increased TRH.
    D. decreased TRH.

68. When N.M. came to see her doctor 10 years ago, which of the following complaints would have been associated with hypothyroidism?
    A. Diarrhea
    B. Jaundice
    C. Protruding eyes (exophthalmos)
    D. Menstrual irregularity

A type 2 diabetic for more than 25 years, C.T. is now nearly 80 years old. His primary health care problems are related to the chronic complications of diabetes.

69. The primary risk factor for type 2 diabetes is:
    A. aging.
    B. obesity.
    C. autoimmune disease.
    D. heredity.

70. In type 2 diabetes, there may be a decreased production of insulin by the β cells of the pancreas, or the pathologic process may involve:
    A. decreased glucagon secretion.
    B. an absolute deficiency of insulin.
    C. increased circulating insulin levels but decreased receptor sensitivity.
    D. antiinsulin antibody formation.

71. Physiologic changes associated with his age, coupled with pathophysiologic alterations related to his diabetes, increase C.T.'s risk for:
    A. hemorrhagic stroke.
    B. osteoporosis.
    C. myocardial infarction.
    D. presbyopia.

72. A condition that contributes to the development of diabetic nephropathy is:
    A. hypertension.
    B. autonomic neuropathy.
    C. renal calculi.
    D. prostate cancer.

73. Which of the following observations is likely associated with a chronic complication of C.T.'s diabetes?
    A. C.T. wears a hearing aid.
    B. C.T. wears glasses to read.
    C. C.T. has partial dentures.
    D. C.T. has a below-the-knee amputation.

P.B. is a 43-year-old electrical engineer. He arrives in the emergency department by ambulance where the paramedics and his wife report a sudden onset of nausea, vomiting, and diarrhea. His blood pressure is very low, and laboratory findings include low blood sugar and profoundly increased serum potassium.

74. This scenario suggests what endocrine emergency?
    A. Thyroid storm
    B. Addisonian crisis
    C. Pheochromocytoma
    D. Diabetic ketoacidosis

75. Appropriate treatment of P.B. requires:
    A. intravenous thyroid hormone replacement.
    B. intravenous insulin administration.
    C. immediate surgery to remove the tumor.
    D. intravenous administration of glucocorticoid.

76. Once he has been treated and routine medications have been established, P.B. should be urged to avoid _____ to decrease the likelihood of recurrence of an emergency.
    A. foods high in carbohydrates
    B. emotional and physical stressors
    C. overdosage of his medication
    D. excessive fluid intake

S.Z. underwent kidney transplantation 3 years ago and has been taking steroids to suppress the immune response and reduce the risk of organ rejection. This medication has produced Cushing syndrome.

77. Although she is only 38 years old, S.Z.'s Cushing syndrome places her at increased risk for what condition that is normally found in people much older than she?
    A. Heart disease
    B. Renal insufficiency
    C. Osteoporosis
    D. Menopause

78. Her blood pressure is carefully monitored because steroids can cause hypertension due to their propensity to cause:
    A. increased contractility of the heart.
    B. atherosclerosis.
    C. sodium and water retention.
    D. increased heart rate.

79. Ecchymoses found on S.Z.'s legs after minor injuries are related to which of the following effects of long-term glucocorticoid administration?
    A. Protein catabolism causing capillary fragility
    B. Increased platelet aggregation
    C. Decreased glucose utilization
    D. Increased glycogenolysis

80. S.Z.'s routine laboratory testing reflects what common finding associated with increased cortisol levels?
    A. Decreased hemoglobin
    B. Increased serum potassium
    C. Decreased BUN
    D. Increased blood sugar

NORMAL ANATOMY AND PHYSIOLOGY REVIEW
Matching

1. D
2. I
3. E
4. B
5. G
6. A
7. L
8. O
9. K
10. P

True/False

11. F
12. T
13. T
14. F
15. T
16. F
17. T
18. T
19. T
20. F

PATHOPHYSIOLOGY QUESTIONS
Fill in the Blank

21. 1
22. polydipsia, polyphagia, polyuria, weight loss
23. acromegaly; pituitary giantism
24. water
25. calcium
26. receptor dysfunction
27. elevated (or increased)
28. exophthalmos
29. surgery
30. muscle atrophy, bone demineralization

Multiple Choice

31. D
32. B
33. A
34. C
35. C
36. B
37. A
38. D
39. D
40. A
41. C
42. D
43. B
44. B
45. A
46. D
47. B
48. D
49. A
50. D
51. A
52. C
53. B
54. C
55. C
56. D
57. A
58. B
59. A
60. C

Case Studies

61. B
62. C
63. A
64. B
65. D
66. C
67. A
68. D
69. B
70. C
71. C
72. A
73. D
74. B
75. D
76. B
77. C
78. C
79. A
80. D

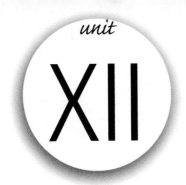

XII Neural Function

Chapters 43 to 47

ANATOMY REVIEW
Matching

1. Match the lettered items in the figure below with the following anatomic terms:

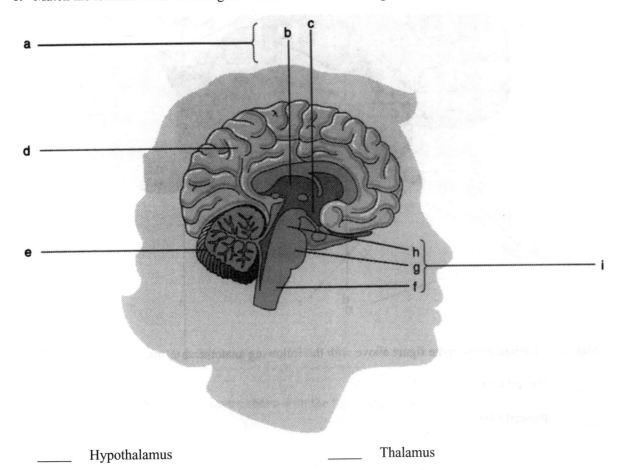

_____ Hypothalamus   _____ Thalamus

_____ Medulla oblongata   _____ Cerebellum

_____ Brainstem   _____ Diencephalon

_____ Cerebrum   _____ Pons

_____ Midbrain

2. Match the lettered items in the figure below with the following anatomic terms:

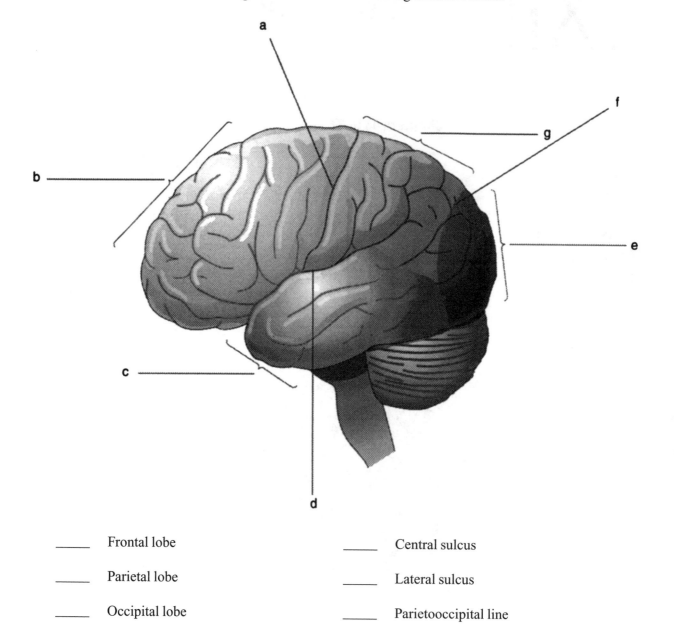

_____ Frontal lobe   _____ Central sulcus

_____ Parietal lobe   _____ Lateral sulcus

_____ Occipital lobe   _____ Parietooccipital line

_____ Temporal lobe

3. Match the lettered items in the figure below with the following anatomic terms:

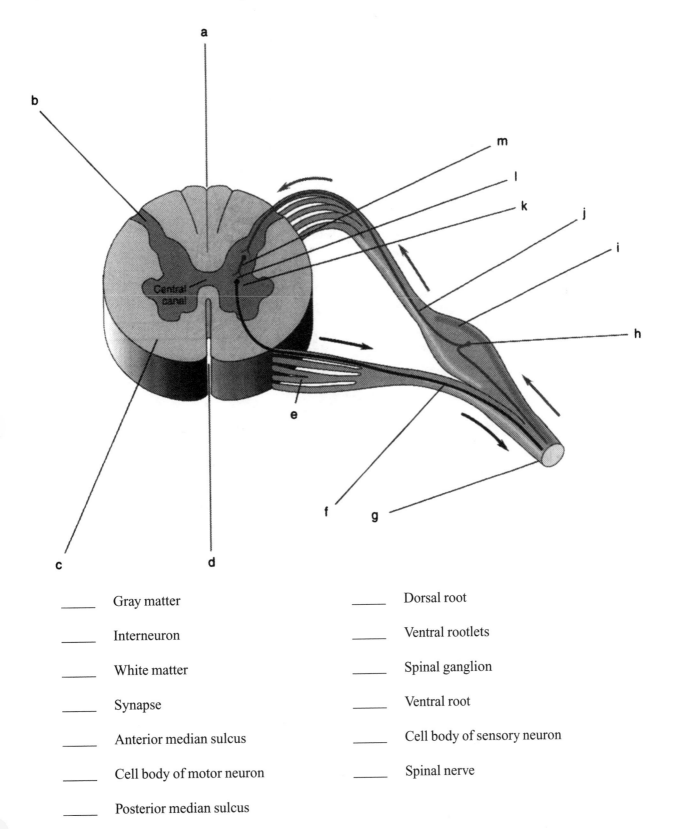

_____ Gray matter

_____ Interneuron

_____ White matter

_____ Synapse

_____ Anterior median sulcus

_____ Cell body of motor neuron

_____ Posterior median sulcus

_____ Dorsal root

_____ Ventral rootlets

_____ Spinal ganglion

_____ Ventral root

_____ Cell body of sensory neuron

_____ Spinal nerve

4. Match the lettered items in the figure below with the following anatomic terms:

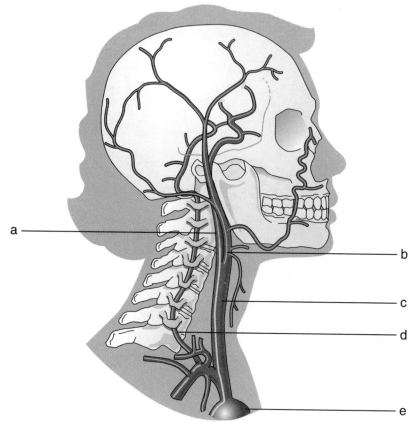

_____ Vertebral artery   _____ External carotid artery

_____ Internal carotid artery   _____ Common carotid artery

_____ Aortic arch

5. Match the lettered items in the figure below with the following anatomic terms:

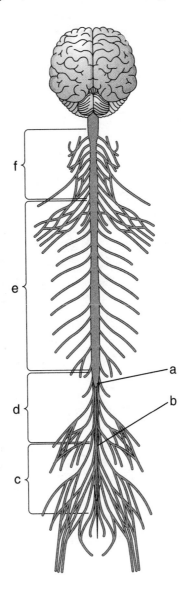

_____ Lumbar segments   _____ Sacral segments

_____ Cauda equina   _____ Conus medullaris

_____ Cervical segments   _____ Thoracic segments

6. Match the lettered items in the figure below with the following anatomic terms:

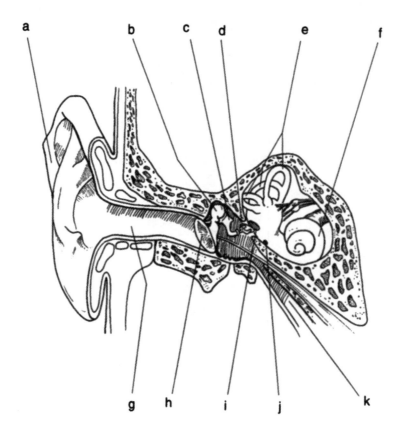

_____ Auricle   _____ Cochlea

_____ Ear canal   _____ Eustachian tube

_____ Incus   _____ Round window

_____ Malleus   _____ Oval window

_____ Stapes   _____ Tympanic membrane

_____ Semicircular canals

7. Match the lettered items in the figure below with the following anatomic terms:

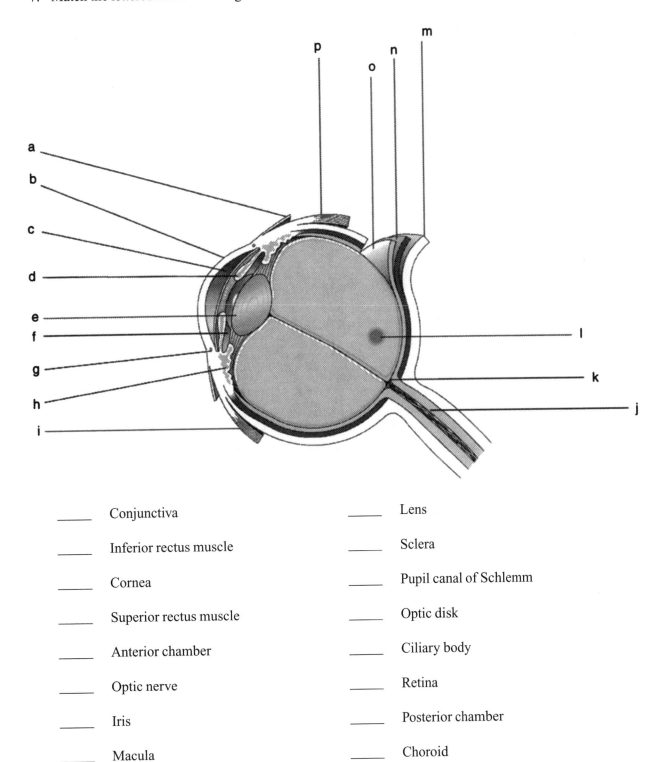

_____ Conjunctiva	_____ Lens
_____ Inferior rectus muscle	_____ Sclera
_____ Cornea	_____ Pupil canal of Schlemm
_____ Superior rectus muscle	_____ Optic disk
_____ Anterior chamber	_____ Ciliary body
_____ Optic nerve	_____ Retina
_____ Iris	_____ Posterior chamber
_____ Macula	_____ Choroid

NORMAL ANATOMY AND PHYSIOLOGY REVIEW
True/False

Indicate whether the following statements regarding the anatomy and physiology of the nervous system are true (T) or false (F).

8. _____ The peripheral nervous system includes 31 pairs of spinal nerves and 12 pairs of cranial nerves.

9. _____ The outermost layer of the brain meninges is the arachnoid.

10. _____ The epidural space lies between the pia mater and the dura mater.

11. _____ Cerebrospinal fluid (CSF) circulates in the subarachnoid space.

12. _____ The sympathetic nerves originate in spinal cord segments T1 through L2.

13. _____ There are two sets of basal ganglia, one in each cerebral hemisphere.

14. _____ The pia mater is adherent to the surface of the brain.

15. _____ The primary motor cortex is located in the parietal lobe.

16. _____ The signal-receiving area of the neuron is the axon.

17. _____ Conduction of action potentials is faster in larger diameter neurons.

18. _____ Glutamate functions as an inhibitory neurotransmitter in the central nervous system (CNS).

19. _____ Excitatory postsynaptic potential results from the opening of potassium and chloride channels in the postsynaptic neuron.

20. _____ Oligodendroglial cells form myelin in the CNS, whereas Schwann cells form myelin in the peripheral nervous system.

21. _____ The primary means of clearing amine neurotransmitters from the synapse is by active reuptake into presynaptic neurons.

22. _____ The thalamus acts as a processor and relay center for both afferent and efferent signals between the cerebral cortex and the brainstem.

Matching

Match the receptors on the left with the correct receptor class on the right. Answers are used more than once.

23. _____ 5-HT$_3$

24. _____ α, β-adrenergic

25. _____ 5-HT$_1$, 5-HT$_2$

26. _____ NMDA

27. _____ nicotinic acetylcholine

28. _____ muscarinic acetylcholine

A. Metabotropic receptor
B. Ionotropic receptor

Match the channel response on the left with the type of postsynaptic potential it generates on the right. Answers are used more than once.

29. _____ Na$^+$ channel opening

30. _____ K$^+$ channel opening

31. _____ Ca^{2+} channel opening

32. _____ Cl$^-$ channel opening

A. Inhibitory postsynaptic potential
B. Excitatory postsynaptic potential

Match each neural structure with its description or function. Answers may be used once or not at all.

33. _____   Anterolateral (spinothalamic) tract

34. _____   Corticospinal tract

35. _____   Dorsal column, medial lemniscal tract

36. _____   Unmyelinated C fibers

37. _____   Myelinated A-δ fibers

38. _____   Occipital lobe

39. _____   Parietal lobe

40. _____   Frontal lobe

41. _____   Temporal lobe

42. _____   Thalamus

43. _____   Microglia

44. _____   Ependymal cells

45. _____   Astrocytes

46. _____   Basal ganglia

47. _____   Extrapyramidal tract

A. Transmit slow pain sensation
B. Transmit fast pain sensation
C. Transmits pain, itch, temperature
D. Transmits fine motor control
E. Transmits fine touch, proprioception
F. Transmits axial motor control
G. Site of primary motor cortex
H. Site of primary somatosensory cortex
I. Site of primary auditory cortex
J. Site of primary visual cortex
K. Structures involved in emotion
L. Relay center of the brain
M. Help maintain blood brain barrier
N. Macrophages of the brain
O. Cells that produce CSF
P. Structures that plan motor programs
Q. Parasympathetic tract

Multiple Choice

Select the one best answer to each of the following questions.

48. Neurons principally communicate through:
    A. action potentials.
    B. chemical synapses.
    C. electrical signals.
    D. gap junctions.

49. The neurotransmitter class of amines includes all of the following neurotransmitters except:
    A. serotonin.
    B. norepinephrine.
    C. dopamine.
    D. acetylcholine.

50. Which of the following neurotransmitters is always inhibitory?
    A. Acetylcholine
    B. Dopamine
    C. GABA
    D. Norepinephrine

51. Inhibitory neurotransmitters produce inhibitory postsynaptic potentials by:
    A. opening voltage-gated sodium channels.
    B. opening ligand-gated sodium channels.
    C. opening chloride or potassium channels.
    D. opening calcium channels.

52. Touch receptors and proprioceptors on the left side of the body:
    A. project to the left somatosensory cortex.
    B. travel up the ipsilateral spinal cord in the dorsal column.
    C. travel up the contralateral spinal cord in the anterolateral column.
    D. cross at the level of entry to the cord and synapse on interneurons.

53. The primary somatosensory and primary motor cortices are:
    A. somatotopically organized.
    B. located in the frontal lobe.
    C. under control of the basal ganglia.
    D. organized into three structural layers.

54. Motor neurons from the corticospinal tract decussate at the:
    A. corpus callosum.
    B. spinal cord.
    C. medullary pyramids.
    D. internal capsule.

55. The principal role of the cerebellum in motor activity is to:
    A. plan the motor program.
    B. activate the α motor neurons in the spinal cord.
    C. improve the match between the intended and actual movement.
    D. provide the motivational force for initiating movement.

56. Deep tendon reflexes are tests of:
    A. spinal cord function.
    B. the monosynaptic stretch reflex.
    C. the Golgi tendon organ.
    D. the flexion withdrawal reflex.

57. REM sleep is associated with:
    A. slow electroencephalographic waves.
    B. dream states.
    C. the most restful type of sleep.
    D. increased muscle tone and motor activity during sleep.

58. The perception of pain can be modulated by endogenous opioids called:
    A. serotonins.
    B. endorphins and enkephalins.
    C. morphines.
    D. catecholamines.

59. Movement of the tympanic membrane in the ear initiates movement of the malleolus, whereas movement of the round window causes movement of the:
    A. stapes.
    B. incus.
    C. perilymph.
    D. hair cells.

60. In the eye, the effect of sympathetic nervous system stimulation is:
    A. contraction of ciliary muscle fibers
    B. pupillary dilation
    C. increased sensitivity of retinal rods
    D. loss of consensual response

Fill in the Blank

Fill in the blanks with the appropriate word or words.

61. Poorly localized pain associated with nausea is transmitted from the receptor to the cord on small, unmyelinated neurons called _____ fibers.

62. Action potentials are usually generated at the initial segment of a neuron because threshold is _____ due to an increased density of _____ _____ _____.

63. The NMDA receptor is a _____ ion channel that binds to the neurotransmitter _____ but will not open unless the membrane is partially depolarized since in the polarized state a _____ ion normally blocks the channel.

64. Glial cells perform many supportive functions in the nervous system, but they do not have voltage-gated ion channels and therefore cannot _____ _____ _____.

65. The six general classes of neurotransmitters are: _____, _____, _____, _____, _____, and _____.

PATHOPHYSIOLOGY QUESTIONS
Multiple Choice

Select the one best answer to each of the following questions.

66. Vertigo commonly occurs with the auditory disorder called:
    A. presbycusis.
    B. otitis media.
    C. Meniere disease.
    D. otosclerosis.

67. Conductive hearing disorders are a result of pathologic lesions of:
    A. the external and middle ear.
    B. the inner ear.
    C. the hair cells.
    D. the vestibulocochlear nerve.

68. Ossification of the bones of the middle ear is an example of:
    A. presbycusis.
    B. conductive abnormality.
    C. sensorineural abnormality.
    D. otitis.

69. Otitis media commonly occurs in children with:
    A. otitis externa.
    B. excessive exposure to loud noise.
    C. foreign body in the ear canal.
    D. eustachian tube dysfunction.

70. An irregular curvature of the cornea or lens results in:
    A. myopia.
    B. hyperopia.
    C. amblyopia.
    D. astigmatism.

71. Patients with diabetes mellitus are at particularly high risk and should be routinely evaluated for:
    A. presbyopia.
    B. vascular retinopathy.
    C. retinal holes and tears.
    D. glaucoma.

72. Which of the following is characteristic of closed-angle glaucoma but not of open-angle glaucoma?
    A. Increased intraocular pressure
    B. Impaired visual acuity
    C. Eye pain
    D. Potential for blindness if untreated

73. A person who experiences a change in olfactory sensation in the absence of an obvious etiologic factor such as cold, inflammation, or smoke inhalation should be evaluated for:
    A. nasal polyps.
    B. brain tumor.
    C. nasal foreign body.
    D. deviation of the nasal septum.

74. The findings of increased blood pressure, pulse, and respiration in a patient are characteristic of pain that is:
    A. chronic.
    B. acute.
    C. referred.
    D. psychogenic.

75. Painful stimulation of visceral structures is often referred to:
    A. the overlying skin.
    B. the gastrointestinal tract.
    C. structures in the same dermatome.
    D. phantom structures.

76. A critical event in determining whether an injured neuronal cell will die is:
    A. rate of action potential conduction.
    B. intracellular calcium overload.
    C. degree of hypoglycemia.
    D. dysfunction of the Na^+-K^+ pump.

77. Hyperventilation to reduce Pa_{CO_2} is likely to produce:
    A. cerebral vasoconstriction.
    B. cerebral hyperoxygenation.
    C. increased cerebral perfusion.
    D. cerebral vasodilation.

78. The brain's normal response to an increase in metabolism or a decrease in arterial perfusion pressure is to:
    A. decrease metabolism.
    B. decrease blood flow.
    C. increase glucose utilization.
    D. vasodilate.

79. A decrease in the size of the cerebral ventricles on computed tomography (CT) scan is indicative of:
    A. hydrocephalus.
    B. increased intracranial pressure (ICP).
    C. subarachnoid hemorrhage.
    D. Alzheimer disease.

80. Normal ICP ranges from:
    A. 0 to 15 mm Hg.
    B. 5 to 25 mm Hg.
    C. 10 to 50 mm Hg.
    D. 25 to 50 mm Hg.

81. The earliest indicator of compromised neurologic functioning is usually:
    A. an altered pupil light reflex.
    B. a change in level of consciousness.
    C. depressed motor responses.
    D. failure to follow commands.

82. The Glasgow Coma Scale has three measures of coma that include all of the following except:
    A. eye opening response.
    B. cognitive processing response.
    C. verbal response.
    D. motor response.

83. Which of the following responses represents the worst neurologic status?
    A. Opens eyes to pain
    B. Withdraws extremity from pain
    C. Wiggles toes to command
    D. Assumes decorticate posture

84. Most head injuries are incurred in:
    A. falls.
    B. motor vehicle accidents.
    C. diving accidents.
    D. sports accidents.

85. Characteristics of epidural hematoma include:
    A. slow progression of bleeding and increased ICP.
    B. venous bleeding from bridging veins.
    C. lucid interval immediately after injury followed by rapid decline in level of consciousness.
    D. extensive primary injury to neuronal structures.

86. The patient most at risk for CNS infection following trauma is one with:
    A. multiple scalp lacerations and abrasions after fall.
    B. a closed head injury after falling off a trampoline.
    C. a basal skull fracture after falling off a ladder.
    D. a laceration of the face and scalp after being hit with a rusty pipe.

87. The most common cause of stroke is:
    A. embolism.
    B. hemorrhage.
    C. thrombosis.
    D. trauma.

88. Patients who experience transient ischemic attacks are at increased risk for:
    A. embolic stroke.
    B. hemorrhagic stroke.
    C. thrombotic stroke.
    D. hypertensive stroke.

89. Which of the following is a significant risk factor for the development of embolic stroke?
    A. Atrial fibrillation
    B. Deep vein thrombosis
    C. Hypertension
    D. Atherosclerosis

90. Typical manifestations of a stroke on the right side of the brain include:
    A. significant aphasia.
    B. weakness on the right side of the body.
    C. loss of vision in the left visual field.
    D. a positive Babinski sign on the right foot.

91. Subarachnoid hemorrhage is most commonly a consequence of:
    A. head trauma.
    B. cerebral aneurysm rupture.
    C. atherosclerotic plaque rupture.
    D. a bleeding disorder.

92. A patient with a headache, stiff neck, fever, and elevated CSF white blood cell count most likely has:
    A. encephalitis.
    B. meningitis.
    C. cerebral abscess.
    D. neuralgia.

93. Seizures are classified as general when they:
    A. are recurrent.
    B. involve both hemispheres of the brain.
    C. produce the same EEG changes.
    D. are preceded by an aura.

94. A patient with dementia and brain atrophy on CT scan or magnetic resonance image is likely to have:
    A. a brain tumor.
    B. a brain infarction.
    C. vascular dementia.
    D. Alzheimer type dementia.

95. Alzheimer disease is associated with a deficiency of brain:
    A. norepinephrine.
    B. dopamine.
    C. serotonin.
    D. acetylcholine.

96. Parkinson disease is associated with a deficiency of basal ganglia:
    A. norepinephrine.
    B. dopamine.
    C. GABA.
    D. acetylcholine.

97. All of the following medications might be appropriate to manage the symptoms of Parkinson disease except:
    A. dopamine precursor (L-dopa).
    B. acetylcholine antagonists.
    C. monoamine oxidase inhibitors.
    D. dopamine receptor antagonist.

98. Clinical manifestations of cerebellar disorders include all of the following except:
    A. ataxia.
    B. intention tremor.
    C. clumsiness.
    D. paralysis.

99. A patient who experiences lower extremity weakness but has normal or increased deep tendon reflexes is likely to have:
    A. multiple sclerosis.
    B. Guillain-Barré syndrome.
    C. spinal shock.
    D. peripheral neuropathy.

100. A congenital anomaly of the spinal cord in which the spinal nerves and meninges protrude from the back is termed:
    A. spina bifida occulta.
    B. meningocele.
    C. myelomeningocele.
    D. spina bifida apparenta.

Fill in the Blank

Fill in the following blanks with the appropriate word or words.

101. The _____ drugs interfere with pain perception in the brain, whereas nociceptor activation is altered peripherally by _____ and _____, and the application of _____ and _____.

102. Symptoms suggestive of TIA are expected to resolve within _____ hours after onset.

103. Myasthenia gravis is a "grave weakness" that worsens with activity, and is due to insufficient amounts of _____ in the myoneural synapse.

104. Intention tremor is indicative of dysfunction of the _____, whereas a tremor at rest is indicative of _____.

105. Most ototoxic drugs affect _____.

106. The two diseases most frequently associated with the development of retinopathy are _____ and _____.

107. Polar primary injury in traumatic brain injury results in damage to opposite sides of the brain due to _____ - _____ movement within the rigid skull.

108. Damage to the Broca area of the brain, most commonly associated with a left-sided stroke, will result in a patient's having difficulty with _____.

109. Although rarely diagnosed in the pediatric population, arteriovenous malformations are vascular abnormalities believed to have a _____ cause.

110. Autonomic dysreflexia is a complication of spinal cord injury that occurs when the _____ nervous system is inappropriately activated below the level of injury, resulting in dangerously elevated _____ _____.

Case Studies

José is a 21-year-old man who was involved in a motorcycle accident and suffered a closed head injury and spinal cord trauma at the cervical 4-5 area. His neck was stabilized in a collar at the scene, and he was flown to the emergency department where he underwent CT. He is unconscious and not responding to verbal commands.

111. Upon admission, a Glasgow Coma Scale assessment is completed. José makes no verbal response, responds to pain by extension (decerebrate posturing), and does not open his eyes to pain. His Glasgow Coma Scale score would be recorded as:
    A. 2.
    B. 3.
    C. 4.
    D. 5.

112. This Glasgow Coma Scale rating indicates:
    A. mild head injury.
    B. moderate head injury.
    C. severe head injury.
    D. brain death.

113. José's CT scan shows a large hematoma in the subdural space. The most likely source of this bleeding is:
    A. middle meningeal artery.
    B. bridging veins.
    C. circle of Willis.
    D. vertebral artery.

114. José is immediately taken to surgery for evacuation of the hematoma and placement of an ICP monitoring device. José's ICP is to be maintained below 25 mm Hg if possible. All of the following measures would be expected to reduce ICP except:
    A. putting the head of the bed down flat.
    B. measures to increase comfort and decrease pain.
    C. mild hyperventilation.
    D. diuretic administration.

115. After his operation José is prophylactically started on antiseizure medications. The main reason for seizure prevention in this case is the fact that seizures:
    A. might compromise the airway and impair respiration.
    B. might cause the intravenous line or ICP monitor to become dislodged.
    C. increase the metabolic activity of the brain and may exacerbate ischemia.
    D. increase the risk of rebleeding of the cerebral hematoma.

116. In the days following his accident José improves markedly. He returns to consciousness and is able to follow motor commands. However, he is unable to move his extremities. He also has bowel and bladder atony, flaccid paralysis, and a loss of spinal cord reflex activity. These findings are consistent with:
    A. autonomic dysreflexia.
    B. spinal shock.
    C. incomplete spinal cord injury.
    D. a good potential for recovery of function.

117. After a few weeks, José's spinal cord reflexes return. José is now at risk for developing autonomic dysreflexia. Signs or symptoms that this problem is occurring would include:
    A. tachycardia.
    B. hypotension.
    C. loss of consciousness.
    D. headache and visual changes.

Mrs. Smith is an 84-year-old resident of a long-term care facility. She has a history of heart failure and is in chronic atrial fibrillation. Her medications include daily aspirin and coumadin. She is normally alert and able to accomplish most of her activities of daily living on her own.

118. This morning Mrs. Smith is still in bed when the aide comes in to check on her. Mrs. Smith is listing to the right side and drooling from the corner of her mouth. She is unable to respond verbally, and the right side of her body is paralyzed. These signs are most likely a consequence of:
    A. right cerebral stroke.
    B. left cerebral stroke.
    C. lacunar stroke.
    D. global hypoxic stroke.

119. The most important consideration during the acute phase of stroke is:
    A. maintaining respiratory and cardiac stability.
    B. determining the location of the stroke.
    C. managing the underlying cause of the stroke.
    D. range of motion to prevent complications.

120. Mrs. Smith is taken to the emergency department where a CT scan is obtained. The purpose of CT at this time is to determine whether the stroke is:
    A. hemorrhagic or ischemic.
    B. in the right or left hemisphere.
    C. large or small.
    D. associated with increased ICP.

121. The CT scan shows that there is no significant intracranial bleeding. Considering Mrs. Smith's history and the CT findings, the cause of her stroke is most likely to be:
    A. embolism.
    B. hypertension.
    C. thrombosis.
    D. hypoxemia.

122. Because of the location of Mrs. Smith's stroke, she is likely to experience:
    A. left-sided neglect.
    B. impaired vision in the left visual field.
    C. aphasia.
    D. altered sensory function in the left side of the face.

Joe is an 88-year-old man with a long history of Parkinson disease. In the last year his family has noticed that his ability to care for himself has deteriorated. He rarely engages in activity and often fails to make it to the bathroom in time. His speech has become progressively more difficult to understand.

123. Joe has been taking L-dopa for many years to manage the symptoms of his Parkinson disease. The drug had worked well for a long time although the dosage had been increased periodically. Joe's family wants to know why he is getting worse instead of better on his medication. Which of the following statements is the best basis for a reply?
    A. L-Dopa helps prevent the progression of Parkinson disease but only partially.
    B. L-Dopa manages the symptoms only and doesn't prevent the continued degeneration that occurs with this disease.
    C. There are much better medications for preventing the progression of Parkinson disease than L-dopa, and Joe should be switched to a different medication.
    D. The decline in Joe's status is probably due to a different process because the L-dopa should continue to work indefinitely.

124. Parkinson disease is associated with:
    A. a deficiency of dopamine in the cerebral cortex.
    B. an overabundance of dopamine in the striatum.
    C. a deficiency of dopamine in the basal ganglia.
    D. a deficiency of acetylcholine in the brain.

125. Sometimes drugs in combination are more effective than L-dopa alone. Which of the following medications would be appropriate to add to Joe's medications to try to improve his motor function?
    A. An anticholinergic agent
    B. A dopamine receptor antagonist
    C. An antipsychotic (haloperidol)
    D. Anticholinesterase

126. Which of the following assessment findings would indicate a positive response to the new drug therapy?
    A. An increase in resistance to passive muscle stretch
    B. An increase in movement of the hands while at rest
    C. A faster, propulsive gait while walking
    D. More frequent swallowing and less drooling

127. Joe's family members ask about the likelihood of inheriting Parkinson disease from their father. Which statement about etiology is the best basis for reply?
    A. Parkinson disease is a familial disorder and family members should be evaluated.
    B. The cause of Parkinson disease is unknown, and no familial pattern has been identified.
    C. Parkinson disease is due to environmental factors only.
    D. Parkinson disease is caused by a virus, and everyone is at approximately equal risk whether they have an affected family member or not.

ANATOMY REVIEW
Matching

1. c, f, i, d, h, b, e, a, g
2. b, g, e, c, a, d, f
3. b, m, c, l, d, k, a, j, e, i, f, h, g
4. d, a, e, b, c
5. d, b, f, c, a, e
6. a, g, c, b, d, e, f, k, j, i, h
7. a, i, b, p, c, j, d, l, e, m, g, k, h, o, f, n

ANATOMY AND PHYSIOLOGY QUESTIONS
True/False

8. T
9. F
10. F
11. T
12. T
13. T
14. T
15. F
16. F
17. T
18. F
19. F
20. T
21. T
22. T

Matching

23. B
24. A
25. A
26. B
27. B
28. A
29. B
30. A
31. B
32. A
33. C
34. D
35. E
36. A
37. B
38. J
39. H
40. G
41. I
42. L
43. N
44. O
45. M
46. P
47. F

Multiple Choice

48. B
49. D
50. C
51. C
52. B
53. A
54. C
55. C
56. B
57. B
58. B
59. C
60. B

Fill in the Blank

61. C
62. low; fast Na^+ channels
63. Ca^{2+}; glutamate; Mg^{2+}
64. generate action potentials
65. acetylcholine; amine; amino acid; neuropeptide; nucleotide; gases

PATHOPHYSIOLOGY QUESTIONS
Multiple Choice

66. C
67. A
68. B
69. D
70. D
71. B
72. C
73. B
74. B
75. C

76. B
77. A
78. D
79. B
80. A
81. B
82. B
83. D
84. B
85. C
86. C
87. C
88. C
89. A
90. C
91. B
92. B
93. B
94. D
95. D
96. B
97. D
98. D
99. A
100. C

Fill in the Blank

101. opioid; prostaglandin inhibitors (NSAIDs), local anesthetics, heat, cold

102. 24
103. Acetylcholine
104. cerebellum; Parkinson disease
105. hair cells of the cochlea
106. hypertension, diabetes mellitus
107. acceleration-deceleration
108. speech
109. congenital
110. sympathetic; blood pressure

Case Studies

111. C
112. C
113. B
114. A
115. C
116. B
117. D
118. B
119. A
120. A
121. A
122. C
123. B
124. C
125. A
126. D
127. B

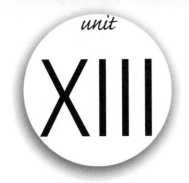

Neuropsychological Function

Chapters 48 to 49

PATHOPHYSIOLOGY QUESTIONS
Fill in the Blank

Fill in the blanks with the appropriate word or words.

1. Although anxiety disorders present with similar manifestations, they differ significantly in terms of the
   _____, _____, and _____ of symptoms.

2. Before an anxiety disorder can be diagnosed, other potential etiologic factors such as _____
   _____ or _____ must be eliminated as the cause of symptoms.

3. Panic disorder is characterized by two types of anxiety behaviors: _____ anxiety and
   _____ anxiety.

4. The significant and pervasive symptom of generalized anxiety disorder is chronic _____ that
   leads to a variety of anxiety symptoms.

5. Comorbid conditions often found to be associated with obsessive-compulsive disorder are
   _____, _____, and _____ _____.

6. Agoraphobia is a rare but debilitating presentation of _____ _____ _____.

7. In severe cases of anorexia nervosa, hypokalemia may result in death from _____
   _____.

8. Recent research findings indicate that abnormalities of _____ _____ are the primary
   biochemical alteration associated with the neuropathologic process of schizophrenia.

9. A person who markedly alters his activities of daily living due to the belief that he is being observed by
   aliens is experiencing _____, whereas a person who proclaims spiders are covering the walls is
   experiencing _____.

10. Depression that lasts 2 or more years but presents with only one or two symptoms is commonly referred
    to as _____ _____ or _____.

Multiple Choice

Select the one best answer to each of the following questions.

11. Psychotic disorders are characterized by:
    A. generalized anxiety.
    B. generalized depression.
    C. altered perceptions of reality.
    D. personality disorder.

12. Nonpsychotic disorders include all of the following except:
    A. schizophrenia.
    B. phobia.
    C. borderline personality.
    D. bulemia.

13. Schizophrenia is usually diagnosed during:
    A. childhood.
    B. adolescence.
    C. young adulthood.
    D. older adulthood.

14. While the cause of schizophrenia is still unknown, all of the following are thought to be associated with its development except:
    A. viral infection during the second trimester of gestation.
    B. genetic predisposition.
    C. unstable childhood.
    D. malnutrition.

15. The "negative" symptoms of schizophrenia are difficult to manage and include:
    A. hallucinations.
    B. disorganized thinking.
    C. delusions.
    D. flat affect.

16. The "positive" symptoms of schizophrenia are attributed to:
    A. excessive stimulation of dopamine (D_2) receptors in the brain.
    B. excessive stimulation of norepinephrine receptors in the brain.
    C. insufficient stimulation of serotonin receptors in the brain.
    D. excessive stimulation of dopamine (D_1) receptors in the brain.

17. Affective disorders are abnormalities of:
    A. personality.
    B. emotion.
    C. reality testing.
    D. social behavior.

18. Major depression is thought to be associated with low brain levels of:
    A. norepinephrine and serotonin.
    B. acetylcholine.
    C. dopamine.
    D. monoamine oxidase.

19. Mania is thought to be associated with a relative excess of brain:
    A. norepinephrine.
    B. dopamine.
    C. acetylcholine.
    D. serotonin.

20. Drugs that may be used to manage depression include all of the following except:
    A. chlorpromazine.
    B. serotonin reuptake inhibitors.
    C. monoamine oxidase inhibitors.
    D. norepinephrine reuptake inhibitors.

21. A patient who experiences periods of reduced sleep and increased activity alternating with periods of low energy and depression is most likely to have:
    A. major depression.
    B. bipolar disorder.
    C. schizophrenia.
    D. delusional disorder.

22. Poor impulse control, increased libido, increased appetite, and grandiosity are characteristics of:
    A. borderline personality.
    B. anxiety disorder.
    C. mania.
    D. schizophrenia.

23. Mania is commonly managed with lithium, a medication that inhibits:
    A. dopamine activity.
    B. norepinephrine and serotonin activity.
    C. norepinephrine receptors.
    D. acetylcholine activity.

24. Tardive dyskinesia is a serious complication of antipsychotic medications characterized by:
    A. hyperthermia.
    B. coma.
    C. involuntary movements.
    D. depression.

25. Anxiety disorders are characterized by:
    A. irrational fears.
    B. poor judgment.
    C. hallucinations.
    D. psychoses.

26. Anxiety disorders include all of the following except:
    A. panic disorder.
    B. delusional disorder.
    C. obsessive-compulsive disorder.
    D. generalized anxiety disorder.

27. A patient who suddenly experiences overwhelming anxiety accompanied by rapid respiration and heartbeat and a sense of impending doom is likely experiencing:
    A. a generalized anxiety episode.
    B. a panic attack.
    C. a severe obsessive episode.
    D. a psychotic break.

28. A person with obsessive-compulsive disorder may feel extremely anxious when:
    A. in unclean environments.
    B. performing the compulsive act.
    C. prevented from performing the compulsive act.
    D. distracted from the obsessive thought.

29. Personality disorders are characterized by:
    A. deviant behavior.
    B. altered perceptions of reality.
    C. depression.
    D. extreme mood swings.

30. A young adult who is excessively possessive of his girlfriend and threatens suicide whenever she attempts to leave him might be diagnosed as having:
    A. depression.
    B. schizophrenia.
    C. borderline personality disorder.
    D. antisocial personality disorder.

31. Lack of anxiety or guilt when doing wrong and a failure to internalize moral and ethical values is characteristic of a person with:
    A. depression.
    B. schizophrenia.
    C. borderline personality disorder.
    D. antisocial personality disorder.

32. Which of the following findings is necessary to apply the diagnosis of anorexia nervosa to a person with an eating disorder?
    A. Female gender
    B. Excessive dietary restrictions
    C. Disturbed body image
    D. Weight loss of more than 15% below appropriate body weight.

33. A major difference between persons with anorexia nervosa and those with bulemia is:
    A. abnormal eating patterns.
    B. episodes of forced vomiting.
    C. concept of body image.
    D. strict dieting.

Case Studies

Sam is a 29-year-old man with a history of alcohol abuse. He is in the clinic today for complaints of fatigue, weight loss, and insomnia.

34. A review of systems reveals that Sam has a long history of low mood with periods when he feels unable to get up in the morning and misses work frequently. He often doesn't feel like eating and may go for several days with minimal intake. He doesn't think there is much point to his life. In view of this history, which of the following diagnoses is most likely?
    A. Bipolar disorder
    B. Anxiety disorder
    C. Depressive disorder
    D. Personality disorder

35. Sam is interested in learning more about the biochemical alterations that contribute to this disorder. An accurate explanation would be that pathogenesis is associated with:
    A. decreased brain serotonin levels.
    B. increased brain norepinephrine levels.
    C. increased activity of D_1 receptors.
    D. increased activity of D_2 receptors.

36. Sam is interested in trying medication to improve his low mood. All of the following medications might be appropriate except:
    A. selective serotonin reuptake inhibitor.
    B. amitriptyline.
    C. serotonin and norepinephrine reuptake inhibitors.
    D. benzodiazepines.

37. After taking his medication for 4 days, Sam calls the clinic to report that it doesn't seem to be helping. Which of the following statements should serve as a basis for reply?
    A. Although side effects may occur rapidly, the mood-elevating effect may take two or more weeks to occur.
    B. The dosage is probably too low and Sam should increase the dose.
    C. This medication is unlikely to be effective, and Sam should be switched to another class of medication.
    D. Sam should keep taking the medication and another medication in a different class should be added.

38. After a month of therapy, Sam is feeling much better. He asks how long he will need to keep taking his medications. Which of the following statements should serve as a basis for reply?
    A. Most patients require only temporary therapy, not lasting more than a month or so.
    B. Many patients will require long-term therapy because of the nature of the biochemical alterations in the brain.
    C. These drugs should be discontinued after 1 or 2 months of therapy because of long-term abuse potential.
    D. Once Sam has been able to stop drinking alcohol, he won't need the medication any longer.

Jane is a 44-year-old woman with a history of mood swings that have become progressively more debilitating over the past several years. She is currently in an "up" mood and feels she is doing fine. However, her husband says he is worried because she is spending a lot of money on various things and is not sleeping at night. Sometimes she won't sleep all night and will have just a short nap in the afternoon. She is otherwise physically well and has no other significant past medical history.

39. Jane would most likely be diagnosed with:
    A. schizophrenia.
    B. seasonal affective disorder.
    C. bipolar disorder.
    D. dysthymia.

40. A biochemical imbalance thought to contribute to mania is:
    A. excessive brain dopamine.
    B. insufficient brain serotonin.
    C. excessive brain norepinephrine.
    D. insufficient brain acetylcholine.

41. A medication traditionally used to stabilize mood swings is:
    A. benzodiazepine.
    B. lithium.
    C. tricyclic antidepressant.
    D. monoamine oxidase inhibitor.

PATHOPHYSIOLOGY QUESTIONS
Fill in the Blank

1. triggers, duration, management
2. physical illness, medications
3. anticipatory, avoidance
4. worry
5. depression, anorexia, Tourette syndrome
6. generalized anxiety disorder
7. cardiac arrhythmias
8. dopamine receptors
9. delusions, hallucinations
10. minor depression, dysthymia

Multiple Choice

11. C
12. A
13. C
14. D
15. D
16. A
17. B
18. A
19. A
20. A
21. B
22. C
23. B
24. C
25. A
26. B
27. B
28. C
29. A
30. C
31. D
32. D
33. C

Case Studies

34. C
35. A
36. D
37. A
38. B
39. C
40. C
41. B

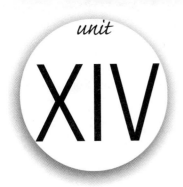

unit
XIV
Musculoskeletal Support and Movement

Chapters 50 to 52

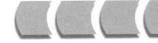

ANATOMY REVIEW
Matching

1. Match each lettered item in the below figure with one of the following anatomic terms:

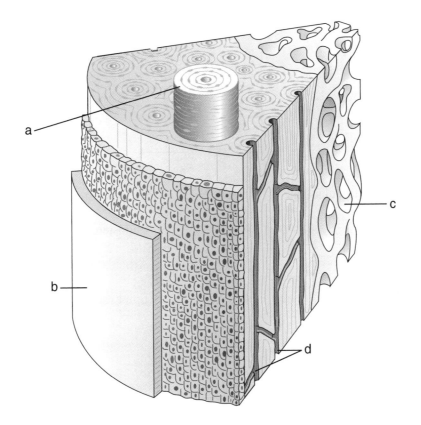

_____ Volkmann canals

_____ Haversian canal system

_____ Periosteum

_____ Cancellous bone

2. Match each lettered item in the figure below with one of the following anatomic terms. Some terms may be used more than once.

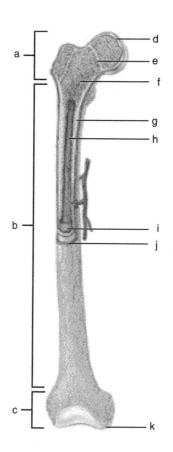

_____ Cancellous/trabecular bone   _____ Periosteum

_____ Epiphysis   _____ Endosteum

_____ Compact/cortical bone   _____ Articular cartilage

_____ Medullary cavity   _____ Epiphyseal line

_____ Diaphysis

NORMAL ANATOMY AND PHYSIOLOGY REVIEW
Matching

Match the terms in the right column with their definitions in the left column.

3. _____ Site of linear growth of long bones.

4. _____ Cells responsible for deposition of bone.

5. _____ Cells responsible for the resorption of bone.

6. _____ Found at the center of each osteon, where blood vessels and nerves are located.

7. _____ Law of bone stresses, which determines deposition and resorption.

8. _____ Stage of fracture healing in which callus is replaced by cancellous/trabecular bone.

9. _____ Movable joints.

10. _____ Located between the tibia and femur, these structures increase weight bearing capacity.

11. _____ Connective tissues that connect muscles to bone.

12. _____ Connective tissues that connect bone to bone.

13. _____ Contractile proteins found in striated muscle.

14. _____ Ion required for muscle contraction.

15. _____ Type of muscle contraction in which no movement occurs.

16. _____ A group of skeletal muscles innervated by a single motor neuron.

17. _____ Energy storage source for muscle contraction.

18. _____ Mature bone cells.

19. _____ Protein found in tendons and ligaments.

20. _____ Immediate source of energy for muscle contraction.

A. Ligaments
B. Consolidation
C. Isometric
D. Adenosine triphosphate
E. Actin and myosin
F. Meniscus
G. Epiphyseal plate
H. Trabeculae
I. Ossification
J. Osteocytes
K. Diarthrodial or synovial
L. Calcium
M. Sarcoplasm
N. Motor unit
O. Osteoblasts
P. Creatine phosphate
Q. Wolff's
R. Tendons
S. Haversian canals
T. Elastin
U. Osteoclasts
V. Glucose

PATHOPHYSIOLOGY QUESTIONS
Compare/Contrast

Compare and contrast rheumatoid arthritis with osteoarthritis by filling in the appropriate columns of the following table with "yes" or "no," indicating the presence of the specific characteristic.

Characteristic	Rheumatoid Arthritis	Osteoarthritis
Systemic manifestations		
Inflammatory disease		
Symmetrical presentation		
Pain at rest		
Laboratory abnormalities		

True/False

Indicate whether the following statements regarding pathophysiology of the musculoskeletal system are true (T) or false (F).

21. _____ All forms of muscular dystrophy have a genetic cause.

22. _____ Infectious arthritis typically involves multiple joints simultaneously.

23. _____ A comminuted fracture is a result of a crushing injury and produces multiple bone fragments.

24. _____ Ankylosing spondylitis causes vertebral fusion.

25. _____ A partial separation of the articulating surfaces of bones within a joint is called a dislocation.

26. _____ Pannus is a vascular scar tissue formed in rheumatoid arthritis that can erode joint tissues and cause contractures.

27. _____ Scoliosis can be detected by observing for uneven alignment of shoulders or hips.

28. _____ Lyme disease is caused by a spirochete whose vector is most often the deer tick.

29. _____ Tuberculosis of bone is a primary form of the disease.

30. _____ Scleroderma manifestations are all due to increased density of the epidermal layer.

Fill in the Blank

Fill in the blanks with the appropriate word or words.

31. CREST is a syndrome associated with scleroderma, where the letters stand for _____, _____ _____, _____ _____, _____, and _____.

32. Acute rheumatic fever is an inflammatory disease that may develop following a throat infection in which the causative organism is _____.

33. _____ fractures are most commonly seen in childhood, when bone is most flexible.

34. Open fractures are classified based on their _____.

35. Contractile tissue injuries (tendons and muscles) are characterized by _____ _____ _____.

36. Defective bone mineralization due to a deficiency of vitamin D in childhood is called _____, whereas its adult counterpart is called _____.

37. Duchenne muscular dystrophy, the most common and severe form, affects only infants and children of the _____ sex.

38. Myasthenic crisis is an acute exacerbation of myasthenia gravis, whereas cholinergic crisis is usually the result of too much _____.

39. The cause of fibromyalgia syndrome is _____.

40. _____, progressing to renal failure, is often found in the multisystem disease known as systemic lupus erythematosus (SLE).

Multiple Choice

Select the one best answer to each of the following questions.

41. Which of the following statements regarding compartment syndrome is true?
    A. A symptom of compartment syndrome is poor muscle tone.
    B. It is due to increased pressure between fascial planes.
    C. It results in impaired fracture healing.
    D. It can be avoided if the fracture is properly aligned.

42. Risk factors for the development of osteoporosis include:
    A. male gender.
    B. African-American race.
    C. decreased weight bearing exercise.
    D. previous fractures.

43. Paget disease differs from osteoporosis in that:
    A. only Paget disease has a hereditary component.
    B. osteoporosis is characterized by excessive and abnormal bone growth.
    C. Paget disease can affect the cranial bones.
    D. osteoporosis primarily affects the long bones.

44. The primary reason osteomyelitis is so difficult to manage is that:
    A. the origin of the infection is usually elsewhere in the body.
    B. antibiotics that are effective against the causative organisms do not exist.
    C. cysts form around the infection.
    D. it is difficult to obtain sufficient antibiotic concentration in bone tissue.

45. The most common malignant tumor of bone is:
    A. osteosarcoma.
    B. Ewing sarcoma.
    C. osteochondroma.
    D. chondrosarcoma.

46. The primary symptom of multiple myeloma is bone pain. This is because:
    A. nerves in bone are more sensitive than those anywhere else in the body.
    B. excessive plasma cell proliferation occurs in the bone marrow.
    C. early metastasis to bone is very common.
    D. as the tumor grows, periosteum is destroyed.

47. A major difference between an injury to a ligament and an injury to a tendon is that:
    A. ligamental injury typically produces decreased muscle strength.
    B. decreased range of motion is common with tendon injury.
    C. passive stretching of an injured ligament will cause pain.
    D. pain is always greater with tendon injuries because more nerve tissue is involved.

48. All muscular dystrophies have in common:
    A. a childhood onset.
    B. a slow onset and progression.
    C. progressive weakness and degeneration of muscles.
    D. the specific muscles that are affected.

49. Which of the following statements regarding myasthenia gravis is true?
    A. It typically presents with weakness of the large muscle groups of the legs.
    B. It is a neuromuscular disease that has its onset in late middle age.
    C. It is due to excessive production of acetylcholinesterase, resulting in decreased amounts of acetylcholine.
    D. It is a progressive autoimmune disease affecting voluntary muscle function.

50. Fibromyalgia syndrome is primarily characterized by:
    A. objective data in the form of specific signs demonstrated by the patient.
    B. emotional instability best managed with psychotherapy and mood-altering drugs.
    C. chronic muscle pain, stiffness, and fatigue.
    D. increased muscle stretch reflexes and muscle spasms.

51. Osteoarthritis:
    A. is an inflammatory disease of the joints.
    B. presents bilaterally in a symmetric distribution.
    C. is characterized by remissions and exacerbations of symptoms.
    D. causes the development of osteophyte spurs.

52. Untreated septic/infectious arthritis may result in:
    A. ankylosis of the joint.
    B. amputation.
    C. prosthetic joint replacement.
    D. septicemia.

53. In addition to affecting diarthrodial joints, rheumatoid arthritis can also affect:
    A. cardiac tissues.
    B. smooth muscle.
    C. ligaments and tendons.
    D. endocrine glands.

54. A characteristic manifestation of SLE that worsens during exacerbations or with exposure to ultraviolet light is:
    A. arthralgia and synovitis.
    B. renal failure.
    C. butterfly facial rash.
    D. pleural effusions.

55. Adults who had acute rheumatic fever as children may come to the hospital because of:
    A. residual joint manifestations.
    B. replacement of a mitral valve.
    C. severe rash resulting in dermal abrasions.
    D. total hip replacement.

56. People prone to developing Lyme disease would be most likely to be exposed while:
    A. rock climbing.
    B. hiking or camping.
    C. water skiing.
    D. down-hill skiing.

57. The underlying pathologic process of gout is:
    A. infection with a bacteria.
    B. painless joint trauma.
    C. muscle injury resulting in myoglobin release.
    D. impaired metabolism of uric acid.

58. Juvenile rheumatoid arthritis:
    A. presents in late adolescence or the early twenties.
    B. is managed with acetaminophen (Tylenol) to reduce inflammation.
    C. differs from rheumatoid arthritis in that there is no systemic involvement.
    D. may disappear once adulthood is reached, but joint damage is irreversible.

59. Patients with rheumatoid arthritis may complain of symptoms of Sjögren syndrome such as:
    A. dryness of the mouth and eyes.
    B. diarrhea.
    C. hypertension.
    D. skin rashes.

60. In the vast majority of patients with rheumatoid arthritis, laboratory testing reveals:
    A. an elevated eosinophil count.
    B. a normal white blood cell count.
    C. a positive rheumatoid factor.
    D. decreased red blood cell sedimentation rate.

61. What is the complication called when a fracture has not healed in 4 to 6 months?
    A. Delayed union
    B. Malunion
    C. Nonunion
    D. Disunion

Case Studies

T.G. is a 58-year-old woman who comes to the clinic for her routine annual physical examination. She says she has been generally in good health this past year, but recently she has noticed increased stiffness in her joints in the morning when she gets up, and some swelling in her knees and wrists. Her nurse practitioner suspects rheumatoid arthritis.

62. In order to meet the criteria for diagnosis of rheumatoid arthritis, additional questions the nurse practitioner might ask could include:
    A. "Have these problems been ongoing for a month?"
    B. "How long does the stiffness last?"
    C. "Have you noticed an increase or decrease in your weight?"
    D. "Have you had any injury to your joints recently?"

63. A diagnostic test result that would be indicative of rheumatoid arthritis would be:
    A. a bone density scan revealing increased porosity of bone.
    B. an x-ray showing joint erosion of the wrists.
    C. rheumatoid factor in the urine.
    D. bacteria in the blood.

64. The joints most commonly affected by rheumatoid arthritis are:
    A. intervertebral joints in the thoracic region.
    B. one of the hip joints.
    C. hands and wrists.
    D. weight-bearing joints.

65. As rheumatoid arthritis advances, a common finding is:
    A. flexion contractures.
    B. pathologic fractures.
    C. pain at rest.
    D. loss of tissue elasticity.

Thirty-five-year-old B.N. has had SLE for the past 5 years. Her treatment currently focuses on supportive interventions and monitoring for the progression of her disease.

66. As an autoimmune disease, the underlying pathologic process of SLE is:
    A. a genetically based hypersensitivity to environmental stimuli.
    B. increased sensitivity to allergens.
    C. deposition of immune complexes in tissues.
    D. an abnormal immune response to infection.

67. The involvement of other organs, and the signs and symptoms associated with their diminished functioning, are associated with:
    A. tissue ischemia and necrosis due to impaired oxygen binding capacity.
    B. calcification of tissues.
    C. invasion of organ basement membranes by immune complexes.
    D. fluid deposition in tissue spaces interfering with nutrient transport.

68. The most common musculoskeletal manifestations of SLE are:
    A. joint pain, swelling, and tenderness.
    B. dislocations and subluxations.
    C. stress fractures.
    D. tendon ruptures and ligamental tears.

K.K. is 76 years old and is healthy for his age. He wears glasses to read and should begin thinking about getting a hearing aid, but his primary complaint is his osteoarthritis. He finds that joint pain is getting in the way of his passion, which is his garden.

69. Osteoarthritis is:
    A. less common than rheumatoid arthritis.
    B. not an inflammatory disease.
    C. involves hand and wrist joints predominantly.
    D. bilateral in presentation.

70. A common finding in the physical examination of a patient with osteoarthritis that is not seen in rheumatoid arthritis is:
    A. joint swelling.
    B. morning joint stiffness.
    C. crepitus with movement.
    D. joint contractures.

71. Interventions that could be beneficial in managing K.K.'s pain could include:
    A. increased weight bearing activities.
    B. steroid therapy.
    C. acetaminophen.
    D. isometric exercises.

R.E. is 10 years old and comes to the Urgent Care Center after taking a fall from his bicycle after his dad tightened his hand brakes. His dad thinks he might have broken his arm. R.E. is otherwise healthy, normal in his growth and development, and has no allergies.

72. Of particular concern when a child breaks a bone is:
    A. a greenstick fracture.
    B. a displaced fracture.
    C. a fracture just below the metaphysis.
    D. a fracture near the epiphyseal plate.

73. An x-ray reveals an oblique fracture of the radius. An oblique fracture is caused by a:
    A. rotational force.
    B. break near the attachment of a ligament.
    C. crushing injury.
    D. demineralization of the bone.

74. R.E.'s fracture is a simple fracture. If it were a compound fracture, a major concern would be:
    A. prolonged healing of the fracture.
    B. infection.
    C. abnormal healing producing deformity.
    D. impaired callus formation.

75. R.E.'s fractured arm is immobilized with a full-length cast. With a new cast and possible continued swelling from the injury, R.E. will be monitored for the development of compartment syndrome. Signs or symptoms of compartment syndrome include all of the following except:
    A. decreased movement of R.E.'s hand and fingers.
    B. hand or fingers are cold to touch.
    C. decreased sensation of hand or fingers.
    D. capillary refill of less than 3 seconds.

Forty-five-year-old W.S. is visiting her physician for her annual checkup. Because her 72-year-old mother has significant osteoporosis, W.S. is asking if there are steps she might take to decrease the likelihood of developing this condition.

76. The underlying pathologic process of osteoporosis is:
    A. increased osteoclastic activity in the face of decreased osteoblastic activity.
    B. loss of cortical bone while cancellous bone remains intact.
    C. increased osteoblastic activity in the face of decreased osteoclastic activity.
    D. collapse of the Haversian canals.

77. Risk factors for osteoporosis in women includes all of following except:
    A. small bone structure.
    B. Caucasian or Asian race.
    C. use of nonsteroidal antiinflammatory drugs.
    D. decreased estrogen following menopause.

78. A patient with significant osteoporosis will likely have:
    A. a decreased serum calcium level.
    B. gingivitis.
    C. decreased height from previous measurements.
    D. decreased muscle stretch reflexes.

79. Prolonged immobility can produce osteoporosis because:
    A. there is increased renal excretion of calcium.
    B. blood flow to the bone is diminished.
    C. parathyroid hormone secretion is decreased.
    D. decreased weight bearing stress impairs osteoblastic activity.

80. Suggestions to W.S. that will decrease the risk for development of osteoporosis include all of the following except:
    A. decreasing alcohol ingestion.
    B. swimming.
    C. hormone replacement therapy at menopause.
    D. walking.

ANATOMY REVIEW
Matching

1. d, a, b, c
2. f, a and c, g, h, b, j, i, d and k, e

NORMAL ANATOMY
AND PHYSIOLOGY REVIEW
Matching

3. G
4. O
5. U
6. S
7. Q

8. I
9. K
10. F
11. R
12. A
13. E
14. L
15. C
16. N
17. P
18. J
19. T
20. D

PATHOPHYSIOLOGY QUESTIONS
Compare/Contrast

Characteristic	Rheumatoid Arthritis	Osteoarthritis
Systemic manifestations	Yes	No
Inflammatory disease	Yes	No
Symmetrical presentation	Yes	No
Pain at rest	Yes	No
Laboratory abnormalities	Yes	No

True/False

21. T
22. F
23. T
24. T
25. F
26. T
27. T
28. T
29. F
30. F

Fill in the Blank

31. calcinosis, Raynaud phenomenon, esophageal hardening, sclerodactyly, telangiectasias
32. β-hemolytic group A *Streptococcus*
33. Greenstick
34. wounds
35. decreased muscle strength

36. rickets; osteomalacia
37. male
38. medication
39. unknown
40. Glomerulonephritis

Multiple Choice

41. B
42. C
43. C
44. D
45. A
46. B
47. C
48. C
49. D
50. C
51. D
52. A

53. A
54. C
55. B
56. B
57. D
58. D
59. A
60. C
61. C

Case Studies

62. B
63. B
64. C
65. A

66. C
67. C
68. A
69. B
70. C
71. C
72. D
73. A
74. B
75. D
76. A
77. C
78. C
79. D
80. B

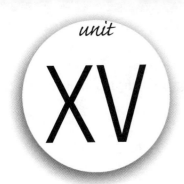
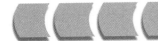

ANATOMY AND PHYSIOLOGY REVIEW
Multiple Choice

Select the one best answer to each of the following questions.

1. The epidermis is composed of:
   A. hair follicles.
   B. nails.
   C. sebaceous and apocrine glands.
   D. stratified squamous epithelium.

2. The predominant cell type in the epidermis is the:
   A. keratinocyte.
   B. basal cell.
   C. histiocyte.
   D. melanocyte.

3. Sebaceous glands are stimulated to produce oil by:
   A. the sympathetic nervous system.
   B. androgenic hormones.
   C. exercise and increased body temperature.
   D. increased skin blood flow.

4. Piloerection is stimulated by:
   A. the sympathetic nervous system.
   B. androgenic hormones.
   C. exercise and increased body temperature.
   D. the parasympathetic nervous system.

5. The primary regulator of skin blood flow is:
   A. the parasympathetic nervous system.
   B. body temperature.
   C. autoregulation.
   D. the baroreceptors.

6. The skin is able to regulate body temperature through increased sweating. Sweating is stimulated by:
   A. the sympathetic nervous system.
   B. the parasympathetic nervous system.
   C. autoregulation.
   D. activation of sebaceous glands.

7. In addition to providing a barrier to microbial invasion, the outer surface film of dead skin cells is important for:
   A. maintaining body temperature.
   B. preventing excessive drying of the skin.
   C. secreting sweat.
   D. sensory perception.

8. Sebaceous glands are most active during:
   A. infancy.
   B. childhood.
   C. adolescence.
   D. adulthood.

9. Young children and the elderly produce less:
   A. sweat.
   B. melanin.
   C. keratin.
   D. nail growth.

10. All of the following changes occur in elder skin except:
    A. thinning of the epidermis.
    B. decreased elasticity of the dermis.
    C. decreased vascularity of the dermis.
    D. increased subcutaneous fat.

11. All of the following are true statements regarding hair loss except:
    A. Baldness is inherited from the mother.
    B. Only men develop recession of the hairline at the forehead.
    C. Hair loss with aging also affects other areas of the body.
    D. Maximal hair distribution occurs at the age of 40, then begins to decline.

12. Changes in the nails associated with aging are primarily due to:
    A. decreased blood flow.
    B. reduced dietary protein.
    C. increased production of keratin.
    D. progressive accumulation of lipofuscin.

PATHOPHYSIOLOGY QUESTIONS
Matching

Match each dermatologic disorder with its correct description. Answers are used only once or not at all.

13. _____ Secondary lesion

14. _____ Macule

15. _____ Papule

16. _____ Nodule

17. _____ Wheal

18. _____ Vesicle

19. _____ Pustule

20. _____ Lichenification

A. Epidermal thickening and rough patches
B. Excessive scar tissue formation.
C. Original appearance, unmodified by time, trauma
D. Lesion has changed from the initial appearance
E. Raised, palpable bump of 0.5 to 2 cm diameter
F. Palpable, circumscribed bump of less than 0.5 cm diameter
G. A blister larger than 0.5 cm diameter
H. Elevated lesion containing purulent exudate
I. A flat, nonpalpable spot up to 1 cm diameter
J. A small blister up to 0.5 cm in diameter
K. An elevated, pink, edematous lesion
L. A thinning of the skin and dermis
M. A collection of serous exudates and debris on the skin

True/False

Indicate whether the following statements regarding the anatomy and physiology of the integumentary system are true (T) or false (F).

21. _____ A primary lesion retains its original appearance, unaffected by time or trauma.

22. _____ The function of skin glands is unchanged by aging.

23. _____ Increased production of melanin with age results in graying of hair.

24. _____ Human papillomaviruses can invade deep into body tissues.

25. _____ Shingles manifests along the dermatomes of the infected sensory nerves.

26. _____ Leprosy is a highly infectious disease caused by a bacterium.

27. _____ Psoriasis can affect individuals of any age.

28. _____ Although acne vulgaris is uncurable, available treatments can be quite effective.

29. _____ Allergic contact dermatitis is a delayed acquired hypersensitivity reaction.

30. _____ Allergic responses to drugs are often apparent as skin manifestations.

Fill in the Blank

Fill in the blanks with the appropriate word or words.

31. _____ _____ is a yeast that causes infections in the throats of newborns and may cause systemic infections in patients who are immunosuppressed.

32. _____ _____ presents as dandruff and cannot be cured, but it can be controlled.

33. In primary syphilis, the ulcerous lesion is called a _____.

34. The most common cause of allergic contact dermatitis is a reaction to _____.

35. Excessive scar tissue is called a _____.

36. Rocky Mountain spotted fever and Lyme disease are both caused by organisms carried by _____.

37. Both topical and systemic _____ may be used in the management of sunburn, depending on severity.

38. In dark-skinned individuals, petechiae may only be visible on the _____ _____ or _____.

Matching

Match each skin disorder with its usual cause. Answers may be used once or not at all.

39. _____ Cold sores

40. _____ Shingles

41. _____ Ringworm (tinea)

42. _____ Impetigo

43. _____ Atopic dermatitis (eczema)

A. Herpes varicella
B. Human papilloma virus
C. Herpes simplex
D. Fungus
E. *Staphylococcus*
F. Allergic reaction
G. Yeast

Multiple Choice

Select the one best answer to each of the following questions.

44. Dark-skinned individuals rarely develop:
    A. alopecia.
    B. basal cell carcinoma.
    C. vitiligo.
    D. seborrheic dermatitis.

45. The underlying pathologic process in the development of pressure ulcers is:
    A. lack of sufficient tissue blood flow.
    B. prolonged immobility.
    C. inadequate nutrition.
    D. profound dehydration.

46. All of the following statements regarding scabies are true except:
    A. The causative organism is a mite.
    B. Scabies is contagious, requiring close personal contact with an affected person.
    C. Scabies is associated with poor personal hygiene.
    D. The predominant symptom is intense itching.

47. Skin manifestations of drug reactions usually include:
    A. a few discrete papules on the extremities.
    B. widespread, pruritic rash.
    C. large halo lesions on the back and trunk.
    D. small, asymptomatic macules.

48. In children, the lesions associated with atopic dermatitis are usually found on:
    A. flexor areas such as antecubital space and behind the knee.
    B. scalp along the hair line.
    C. the hands and between finger webs.
    D. palms of hands and soles of feet.

49. Which of the following neoplastic disorders of the skin carries the worst prognosis?
    A. Basal cell carcinoma
    B. Squamous cell carcinoma
    C. Melanoma
    D. Senile keratoses

50. *Vitiligo* is a term that describes:
    A. a patch of skin with excessive fine hair growth.
    B. a depigmented patch of skin.
    C. a hyperpigmented area of skin.
    D. a lichenified area of skin.

51. Pallor is best assessed by examining nail beds, lips, and:
    A. underside of the tongue.
    B. palms of the hands.
    C. earlobes.
    D. conjunctiva.

52. Often associated with repeated insulin injections, lipodystrophies appear as:
    A. raised, palpable nodules.
    B. areas of hyperpigmentation.
    C. smooth, large depressions.
    D. rough, thickened areas.

53. Excessive hair growth is:
    A. associated with excessive estrogen.
    B. common in Native Americans.
    C. called "hirsutism."
    D. indicative of increased peripheral circulation.

54. Spoon nails commonly are a manifestation of:
    A. iron deficiency anemia.
    B. chronic hypoxemia.
    C. an episode of high fever.
    D. heart failure.

55. Immunization is not available for:
    A. rubella.
    B. measles.
    C. chickenpox.
    D. roseola.

56. Children who present with skin rashes accompanied by fever are most likely experiencing:
    A. parasitic skin infestation.
    B. viral infection.
    C. allergic skin reaction.
    D. idiopathic skin reaction.

57. The most common burn injury in children, accounting for 60% of all burns in children younger than 15 years, is:
    A. electric shock injuries.
    B. external chemical burns.
    C. scald injuries.
    D. exposure to flame.

58. Second-degree burns involve the:
    A. epidermis only.
    B. epidermis and dermis.
    C. epidermis, dermis, and subcutaneous tissue.
    D. epidermis, dermis, subcutaneous tissue, and underlying muscle and bone.

59. Third-degree burns involve the:
    A. epidermis only.
    B. epidermis and dermis.
    C. epidermis, dermis, and subcutaneous tissue.
    D. epidermis, dermis, subcutaneous tissue, and underlying muscle and bone.

60. A burn is classified as major if it covers more than:
    A. 10% of the body surface of a child.
    B. 15% of the body surface of an adult.
    C. 20% of the body surface of a child or adult.
    D. 25% of the body surface of an adult.

61. The best way to extinguish flames on a burning individual is by:
    A. dousing the flames with water.
    B. rolling the person on the ground.
    C. smothering the flames with a blanket or cover.
    D. using a standard fire extinguisher.

62. Major burns are commonly associated with burn shock in which there is:
    A. excessive edema and fluid volume overload.
    B. significant hemorrhage and anemia.
    C. massive capillary leakage and volume deficit.
    D. rapidly developing sepsis.

63. Topical rather than systemic antibiotics are the preferred treatment for burn injury because:
    A. the infecting organisms are entering through the skin.
    B. the burned area is poorly vascularized.
    C. the required antibiotics are available only in topical form.
    D. intravenous access is difficult to establish.

Case Studies

B.N. is a 9-year-old girl brought to the clinic by her mother for evaluation of an itchy skin rash. There is no significant medical history and no known allergy. A review of systems reveals only that B.N. reacts excessively to mosquito and other bug bites, which sometimes cause swelling of the lips and face; however, there has never been any respiratory difficulty associated with these reactions.

64. The skin lesions show evidence of chronic scratching and are thickened and scaly. These lesions would be classified as:
    A. primary lesions.
    B. secondary lesions.
    C. macules.
    D. papules.

65. The physical assessment findings indicate probable eczema. In assessing the skin, the nurse is aware that the location especially likely to have lesions in this disorder is:
    A. behind the knee.
    B. around the ankles.
    C. on the shoulders.
    D. on the scalp.

66. In addition to topical corticosteroids, an important therapy for eczema is:
    A. application of drying gels.
    B. frequent bathing in very warm water.
    C. frequent application of skin moisturizers.
    D. application of occlusive dressings.

67. B.N. asks what is causing the itchy rash. Which of the following statements is the best basis for a reply?
    A. The cause of eczema is unknown.
    B. Eczema is thought to be a kind of allergic reaction.
    C. Eczema is secondary to a nervous habit of frequent scratching.
    D. Eczema is simply a dry skin condition.

68. B.N.'s mother is concerned that the topical corticosteroid might have dangerous side effects. Which of the following statements is the best basis for a reply?
    A. The side effects of topical corticosteroids are similar to those of oral corticosteroids.
    B. When used as prescribed, topical corticosteroids have minimal systemic effects.
    C. The only side effect of topical corticosteroids is thinning of the skin.
    D. Topical corticosteroids can only be used for one week to avoid serious side effects.

69. Itching (pruritus) is the most disturbing feature of eczema (atopic dermatitis). Should the usual interventions be unsuccessful, which of the following systemic treatments should be ordered?
    A. Antihistamines
    B. Antibiotics
    C. Steroids
    D. Barbiturates

C.Y. is a 6-year-old boy who suffered a scald injury on his arm and chest when he fell into a bathtub that was filling with hot water. His parents quickly submerged the burned area in cold water and then brought him to the emergency department.

70. Upon arrival at the emergency department, C.Y. is crying and says the burned area is painful. The skin is blistered in several areas and the skin is sloughing in others. The burn is categorized as second degree. This means that:
    A. only the epidermis is damaged.
    B. only the epidermis and dermis are damaged.
    C. the epidermis, dermis, and subcutaneous tissue are damaged.
    D. the sensory receptors in the skin have been destroyed.

71. The burn is estimated to cover about 10% of the total body surface area. This means that the risk for burn shock is:
    A. high.
    B. low.

72. The parents are concerned about whether they did the right thing in submerging C.Y. in cold water after the burn. Which of the following is the best reply for the nurse to make?
    A. "Yes, cold water is a good way to decrease the pain, although it may not reduce the degree of burn."
    B. "Yes, cold water is the best way to extinguish a burn and reduce the degree of burn."
    C. "No, simply applying wet cloth to the burn would avoid damage to the burned area."
    D. "No, tepid water would be more effective and less of a shock to the skin."

73. C.Y.'s parents are instructed to apply Silvadene to the burn twice daily and to observe for signs and symptoms of infection. They are told to seek medical attention in the event of:
    A. failure of the burn to heal within a week.
    B. oozing of serous fluid from the blistered areas.
    C. sloughing of skin from burned areas.
    D. progressive swelling and redness of the skin surrounding the burn.

NORMAL ANATOMY AND PHYSIOLOGY
Multiple Choice

1. D
2. A
3. B
4. A
5. B
6. A
7. B
8. C
9. A
10. D
11. B
12. A

PATHOPHYSIOLOGY QUESTIONS
Matching

13. D
14. I
15. F
16. E
17. K
18. J
19. H
20. A

True/False

21. T
22. F
23. F
24. F
25. T
26. F
27. T
28. T
29. T
30. T

Fill in the Blank

31. *Candida albicans*
32. Seborrheic dermatitis
33. chancre
34. plants
35. keloid
36. ticks
37. steroids
38. oral mucosa; conjunctiva

Matching

39. C
40. A
41. D
42. E
43. F

Multiple Choice

44. B
45. A
46. C
47. B
48. A
49. C
50. B
51. D
52. C
53. C
54. A
55. D
56. B
57. C
58. B
59. C
60. D
61. A
62. C
63. B

Case Studies

64. B
65. A
66. C
67. B
68. B
69. A
70. B
71. B
72. B
73. D